7 Fat Loss Facts After 40

How to Lose Weight and Feel Great in Less Than a Week

By Dr. Amanda Borre, D.C.

Table of Contents

A Little Bit About It

My name is Dr. Amanda Borre, D.C., and I'm a mother, daughter, sister, and friend—wearing all of the hats, just like you. I've been helping people become healthier for decades, but the year 2015 was when I really began to zero in on weight-loss issues. I made the switch after seeing that the majority of my overweight female patients were over the age of 40. Now, I'm no stranger to gaining weight and have fought with similar issues in the past, which is why I didn't want the secrets of reducing weight after 40 to be accessible exclusively to those who come to see me in person. In order to provide you with the knowledge in this book, I spent a considerable amount of time doing further research from books, the internet, medical publications, my own personal knowledge, and even my own patients. Because I am patient-obsessed and I enjoy seeing progress, this kind of activity is my absolute passion.

Over the years, I have assisted thousands of people in losing weight, and the reason I have such a high success rate is because I look at each client as an individual and provide them with 1:1 care according to their specific needs. Here, I will be able to give you general knowledge that has worked for the majority of patients. If you want the 1:1 concierge care, just reach out and I would be happy to provide that remotely-anywhere-for you as well. I always try to have an open mind, and I believe I have researched and heard of almost every kind of diet, fad or not, in my clinic. I actually test most anything I hear about myself because I want to give honest feedback when patients ask about other programs. I'd rather test them myself in my clinic because I never want to see any of my patients put their health in danger for a fad diet that might end up doing them more damage in the future. One thing I've learned from all these fad diets is that they don't work in the long run. If you want to lose weight for good, ladies, just keep reading.

Introduction

Ever wonder why those old diet tricks just aren't cutting it anymore? In your 20s and 30s, you could skip a meal here or there or put in some extra time at the gym, and the weight came right off—but not anymore! This is due to the fact that maintaining a healthy weight is harder for our bodies as we get older. This irritating problem affects most women, if not all. You may have seen actress Charlize Theron's recent portrayal of infamous serial murderer Aileen Wuornos in the movie, *Monsters*, or if not, you probably at least know who she is. This amazing actress has a history of changing her physical appearance to play different roles, as shown in *Monsters*, but for her role in another of her greats, *Tully* she really upped the ante. Theron portrays Marlo, a lady who is about to give birth to her third child and is also at risk of developing postpartum depression. This is, however, before her brother sends her an evening nanny called Tully to assist her. Therefore, the usually gorgeous and athletic Charlize Theron—who in real life is a loving mother of two children via adoption—had to put on 50 pounds in order to represent a postnatal figure that was really authentic. Despite the fact that in the past she could more readily put on weight and take it off for previous movie roles, Theron, who was 42 at the time, noted that losing the weight she put on for the role took a lot longer at that age, than it did when she was in her twenties. "Losing that weight took me a year and a half," she said in an interview with (Garcia-Navarro, 2018). "Women do this every day, yet it was one of the worst things my body went through." And she is right; the challenges that women encounter every day do not get nearly enough attention.

Being at this stage can be extremely stressful. It's easy to wonder why your body is suddenly not functioning as it once did. To make things worse, it's also easy to get overwhelmed with different programs that make weight loss promises, leaving you even more perplexed about the best course of action. Are you sick and tired of all the information and just want to know a simple, fast, and well-proven strategy to reduce weight right now? Trust me, I understand; not only as a woman who has researched this topic avidly for quite some time but also as one who has struggled myself, I can confidently state that you've chosen the proper book! In it, I explain why it's more difficult for women over 40 to lose weight and keep it off, as well as how to solve this and lose weight in under a week. I know it seems a bit far-fetched at first, but I promise it will make a lot more sense as you read on.

Why This Is the Right Book for You

Many women find it much more difficult to lose weight once they reach the age of 40 and are perplexed as to why. All of a sudden, the weight-loss strategies they had relied on in the past stopped working. I understand because I've treated a lot of patients like this; in fact, before I discovered the best approach for me and my patients, I went through the same experience. Our bodies change as we age due to a variety of factors, including hormones, stress, and muscle loss, which leads to the accumulation of fat (especially around our belly area). Because of this, I've compiled the most crucial knowledge that will not only show you how to lose weight and keep it off but also lend some answers as to why. After all, it's impossible to begin addressing your weight and health problems after you hit 40 unless you have a firm grasp on the ways in which your body has changed. This book is not about magic cures or fast remedies since, surprise! There are none. If you are serious about losing weight and keeping it off, you will need to put in some effort, but that does not always mean working harder. I will demonstrate how you can work more efficiently to get the results you want in half the time. Imagine if there was a book that showed you how to lose weight without having to do hours of aerobics every day and without always feeling hungry. Well, you're in luck then, because you've just picked up such a book!

Here we go into detail on how water may be your greatest friend when it comes to having glowing skin and rapid weight loss, how your habits can cause you to gain weight unknowingly and what you can do to stop it, how to get rid of constipation and so much more! I've been accused of being too optimistic (and this book will undoubtedly reflect that), but I don't know how else to be after witnessing the outcomes my patients and I have had after following the advice I provide in the following facts. No matter how unsuccessful your previous efforts at weight loss have been, chances are they just weren't the right match for you, or maybe you weren't provided with enough information. In any case, being a Debbie downer won't help you much. Instead, I think that if you remain upbeat and keep trying, you'll eventually succeed. Add to that a realistic plan, and that weight could start coming off in less than a week. Even though we can't stop getting older and it's just a natural part of life, we don't have to "feel" old. Self-confidence is important at any age, and making yourself appear the way you want to is a great place to start. I'm a straightforward gal who thinks that good advice should be useful, instructive, and easy to implement. With the help of this book, you can start right now to look and feel better, lose weight more quickly, and improve your overall health.

Fact 1:

Why Water?

We all know that the saying "Water is life" is more than just a cliche. Besides helping us stay alive, this "drink of life" can actually help us on our weight-loss journey if we're willing to make it our new best friend. While I can't guarantee that chugging a glass of water before bed will cause you to magically lose weight the next morning, there is evidence to suggest that it may help. Water is necessary for every bodily function, which should come as no surprise given that it makes up approximately 60% of the human body. According to research, the more hydrated you are when engaging in tasks like thinking and fat burning, the better your body will perform. For the sake of your general health, it's crucial that you drink enough water each day. By drinking enough water, you may avoid being dehydrated, which can hurt your memory, change your mood, make your body overheat, and cause constipation and kidney stones. Water also has no calories, so drinking it instead of drinks with calories, like sweet tea or sugary soda, can help you control your weight and eat less.

Why Increasing Your Water Intake Aids in Weight Loss:

1. **Water has the ability to naturally reduce your hunger**

   When hunger strikes, your first inclination may be to go for food, but this isn't always the smartest move -or what your body needs. The brain often misinterprets thirst, which is caused by even moderate dehydration, such as hunger. This means that if you are low in water, not food, drinking water may help you feel full. This is why drinking water right before your meal may help you eat less as well. Just think about it for a minute. If, say, drinking two glasses of water makes you feel full, then you will naturally eat less because you are less hungry. (Corney et al., 2015) showed in a small 2015 study that individuals who drank two glasses of water just before a meal ate 22% less than those who did not drink any water before eating. Two glasses of water should be enough to fill your stomach until your brain recognizes fullness. (Davy et al., 2008) performed another trial in which middle-aged overweight and obese volunteers lost 44% more weight when they drank water before each meal than when they did not. The same study also found that drinking water before breakfast cut the number of calories consumed. It's important to note that research on younger people hasn't shown the same dramatic drop in calorie consumption, but middle-aged and older people may benefit a lot more from this.

2. **Water May Help to Boost Your Metabolism**

Drinking water may help your body burn more calories and speed up its metabolism, which can help you control your weight. In fact, to prove this, a study published by (Vij, 2013) in The Journal of Clinical and Diagnostic Research found that the body mass index and body composition scores of 50 overweight women went down when they drank two cups of water half an hour before each meal for eight weeks. The study's objective was to determine if excessive water consumption helped overweight participants lose weight and body fat. At its conclusion, the research essentially acknowledged and showed the significance of water-induced thermogenesis for the weight loss of obese individuals. Burning calories, or thermogenesis, is a metabolic process that organisms use to create heat. In other words, thermogenesis is the process through which the body "burns" calories to produce heat.

This is not a feat of magic: Water, particularly cold water, seems to boost thermogenesis in the human body. The body must use energy to get the fluid to body temperature; the more energy you burn, the faster your metabolism (the system through which your body converts food and liquids into energy) functions. In a tiny study by (Boschmann et al., 2003) 14 healthy people drank two cups of 71°F water, and their metabolism increased by 30% on average. Before you fill your glass and still over-pile your plate, you should know that the benefits of thermogenesis probably won't cause you to burn a LOT of calories and lose weight. Because drinking more water has few, if any, negative consequences, it is still important to stay hydrated-even if the impact is minor.

3. **Drinking More Water Can Help You Consume Fewer Liquid Calories Overall**

Because water does not have any calories, drinking it instead of other higher-calorie options like juice, soda, sweetened tea or coffee is one way to cut down on the total number of calories you consume via liquids. Drinking water instead of the typical 20-ounce soft drink from the vending machine can save you 250 calories. The calorie savings may build up rapidly as long as you don't "make up" for those calories, i.e., leave the coffee shop with a bagel and water instead of your typical flavored cappuccino. It's also important to note that although diet soda has no calories, switching to water instead of diet drinks will still help some individuals lose weight. In a study by (Madjd et al., 2015) overweight and obese women who switched from diet drinks to water after their main meal lost more weight while on a weight-loss program. The greater weight reduction in individuals who drank water might be linked to ingesting fewer calories and carbs, according to the researchers, but further study is required.

4. **Hydration Is Especially Important While Working Out**

During exercise, the body needs water because it dissolves and distributes electrolytes, which are minerals like sodium, potassium, and magnesium that cause the muscles to contract in order to move the body. One of the signs of an electrolyte imbalance, which can happen if you don't drink enough, is cramping. You won't get as much out of your exercises if you don't drink enough water before and throughout your workouts since dehydrated muscle cells break down protein (muscle) more rapidly and develop muscle slower.

During exercise, the body also loses fluids more quickly because it generates heat. This heat is transferred to the surface of the skin, where sweating and evaporation, a cooling process, help keep the body at a comfortable temperature. Maintaining a healthy level of hydration helps keep your blood volume steady, which in turn lets your blood vessels at the surface of your skin expand as much as possible, which helps release heat. If your body can't get rid of too much heat through sweating, you could get heat exhaustion. Hydration may help you get more out of your workout and even your day overall, whether it's by keeping you alert or by helping you stay active for longer. Rather than waiting until you're thirsty, it's important to drink water before, during, and after your workout.

5. **Water Helps Get Rid of Body Waste**

Because water makes up a large portion of urine and because water keeps stools soft, drinking water makes it easier to produce urine and move your bowels. So, if you drink enough water, your digestive system will have an easier time moving things along, and you won't have to worry as much about gas and constipation. Keeping yourself hydrated is also important for maintaining healthy kidney function, getting rid of any germs that may have settled in your urinary system, and avoiding the formation of kidney stones due to too concentrated urine.

6. **Hydration helps boost and sharpen attention**

Fatigue, dizziness, and disorientation are all indicators of dehydration, and who makes good choices when they're feeling like that? Certainly not me! Sleepiness and decreased attentiveness may also be caused by dehydration. Dehydration boosts your body's production of cortisol, the stress hormone. According to a research study published by (Castro-Sepulveda et al., 2018), if you experience any of these symptoms, it may be time to increase your water intake and make some healthier eating choices.

7. **For the body to burn fat, it needs water**

If you don't drink enough water, your body may have a hard time breaking down your stored fat and carbohydrates. This is due to the fact that dehydration results in a decrease in lipolysis inside the body. Lipolysis, which may be brought on by hormonal changes, is the process of breaking down fat to provide energy for the body. (Thornton, 2016) describes how an increase in lipolysis resulted in more weight loss for his subjects in a blog post. Because of this, it is essential to consume an adequate amount of water if you really want to rid your body of the fat that you eat as well as the fat that you store. Not to mention, you also burn more calories at rest when you drink water. This is called resting energy expenditure. Within 10 minutes of consuming water, humans have a 24-30% spike in their resting energy expenditure, which should last for at least an hour. In support of this, research conducted on overweight and obese children and published by (Brown et al., 2006) indicated that their REE increased by 25% after drinking cold water.

In yet another study, participants who were overweight women were asked to increase their water intake to more than one liter (or 34 ounces) each day. The purpose of this study was to explore the consequences of doing so. Also (Stookey et al., 2008) found that this led to an additional loss of 2 kilograms (4.4 lbs) in body weight over the course of a year. These results are very astounding given that the only change these women made to their daily routine was to drink more water. The participants in each study also discovered that drinking 0.5 liters (17 oz) of water resulted in an extra 23 calories burned. That's enough to make you gain more than 2 kilograms (4.4 pounds) of fat in a year, which is about 17,000 calories. When the water is cold, your body expends even more calories in order to warm it up to body temperature, so the colder it is, the better!

8. **Becoming Hydrated and Slim—How Much Water Should You Drink?**

Imagine being on the best diet for weight loss and still not being able to lose weight fast enough. My buddy Claire experienced this. Even though Claire was exercising four times a week and eating healthily, she was still losing much less weight than she had anticipated in the time frame she had set for herself. She was starting to lose motivation and didn't believe she would ever get to her ideal weight. She admitted to me that she had even considered stopping her morning runs since she often felt lightheaded and disoriented when she tried to push herself over greater distances. The fact that she was a mother to two young boys who kept her rather busy added an extra challenge.

After listening to her, I asked her if she was drinking enough water because she couldn't figure out what she was doing wrong. Yes, she said quickly, but when she thought about it more, she had to admit that her water use had been very random. She said, "I don't always remember to drink water during the day; sometimes I simply drink my coffee." I could absolutely believe it, being a busy mom myself. We often just don't take the time to take care of ourselves or assess simple things like drinking water as a measure of self-care. I explained that because our bodies are mostly water, they need proper hydration to truly thrive. She began to realize that even if she ate the "perfect" diet, she wouldn't lose weight because dehydration makes it impossible for the body to burn fat. But first and foremost, what does it even mean to say that someone is "fully hydrated"? Well, a daily intake of eight 8-ounce glasses of water (or roughly 2 liters) is what is recommended by most health experts. This number is, however, absolutely arbitrary.

The amount of water an individual needs to drink, like so many other things, is totally dependent on the person. Those who are very active, for example, may require more water than those who are not. It is also critical for older people and nursing mothers to monitor their fluid intake. As a general guideline, strive to drink between 0.5 and 1 ounce of water per pound of body weight every day. The basic rule for calculating this is to split your body weight in half. So, if you weigh 200 pounds and do exercise that isn't too hard, you should drink 100 ounces of water. If you want to exercise or go on a track, you should add to those 100 ounces. You should drink 12 ounces of water two hours before your workout and another 12 ounces 30 minutes before it starts. Of course, you should drink during the activities. When figuring out how much water you should consume, you may also want to think about your environment and any illnesses or health problems you have. When it's hot or humid outdoors, you will sweat more and thus need to drink more water. If you are sick, vomiting, or have a fever, you will lose fluid more quickly and will need to rehydrate.

Get a Fun, Pretty Cup So You Like It

Okay, so you know by now that drinking water is basically a necessity if you want to lose weight, but I know that sometimes it can be really hard to consume the recommended 1/2 oz per 1lb of body weight daily. It's very easy to get caught up in your day and forget to drink enough water, which is why carrying a reusable water bottle is always a smart idea. It's much more convenient to have a refillable water bottle on hand when you're out and about, on the road, at your desk, at home, or at your children's school. A water bottle may also act as a sort of visual reminder for you to drink more water if it is kept nearby. Try leaving the bottle on your work desk or anywhere where you spend a lot of time. This continual visual cue will encourage you to drink more water.

Many popular dietitians and coaches who help people lose weight recommend this refillable water method! In fact, registered dietitian Monica Auslander said that carrying water makes you drink more because of the exposure effect (Quinn, 2016). As a psychological phenomenon, the "mere-exposure effect" describes how individuals like something just because they are used to seeing it. It also goes by the name of the "familiarity principle" because of this. Another bonus to this is that the planet will thank you since reusable bottles are also more eco-friendly than using plastic water bottles, which can only be used once. Carrying and using a water bottle that can be used more than once also demonstrates that you are conscientious about the environment and that you are an astute shopper.

One fun way to get more water is to customize your water bottle as you like, which is great for displaying your individuality and creating a fashion statement everywhere you go. What I'm about to say may seem completely out there, but I've found that having a nice water bottle or cup to sip from makes me more likely to keep up with my water intake and push myself a little farther during workouts. And I'm not alone in feeling this way. We all know that humans are drawn to visually beautiful objects, so if you're going to be lugging around a water bottle all day, it might as well be one you like looking at. I guess knowing that our water bottle looks good and makes us look good gives us a little extra motivation, and who doesn't want to look good?

Use a Straw for Easy Access

Straws have been used by humans for thousands of years. The straw has been around since at least 3000 B.C., but at that time, Sumerians used gold tubes to sip on their beers. In the 1800s, straws were made out of rye stalks. Even though the paper straw was invented in 1888, most people didn't start using plastic straws until the 1970s. Straws are commonly used nowadays. Every day, between 170 million and 490 million plastic straws are used in the United States alone. Reusable straws come with most Starbucks or Yeti cups or can be purchased cheaply to go with any mug, tumbler, or cup. They wash easily and are easier on the environment too! Straws also make it easier for those with impairments to drink beverages safely.

However, another benefit you might be surprised to hear about is that straws are actually better for increasing hydration than drinking straight from a cup or bottle. I think most people would expect the reverse, but for some reason, using a straw allows you to consume more water in a shorter period of time. Specialists themselves aren't quite sure why we drink more fluids when we use a straw, but one potential reason is that because it's easier to drink with a straw, we drink more without even realizing it.

Straws make it possible to stay hydrated when working on the computer or reading a book without always having to remove the lid. It helps you do more than one thing at once, and it can become a habit that you do without thinking.

I tried this for myself; for two weeks, I sipped all my beverages with a straw. I was surprised to discover that I had consumed more water than usual. I also got similar stories from my patients. Straws aren't for everyone, but I think you'd benefit from giving them a try for a week or so and seeing how you like them. If you're still not convinced, try drinking from a bottle or cup without a straw and then from one with a straw to see if you notice a difference. Be careful when you decide to use a straw with all your drinks because if you're sipping on a high-sugar beverage, it can be easy to gain unwanted weight. Also, be careful with alcoholic beverages since you might become drunk without even meaning to.

Fact 2:

Diet Diaries

Though it's true that drinking water can help you limit your food intake, it won't do you much good if you're still eating too much or the wrong sorts of food, even if you're drinking enough water. You'll probably not reach your weight-loss goals as fast as you'd like, if at all, depending on what you eat. That's where a food diary can be handy. A food diary allows you to keep track of what you eat and how much you eat in a day. It's easy to overeat during the day, with mindless snacking, busy schedules, chewing sugary gum, etc. Therefore, a food diary can be a very helpful tool for those who want to start taking charge of their eating habits. Tracking what you eat may shed light on your eating routines and habits and reveal your go-to meals, both healthy and otherwise. Keeping a diary has been shown to be a useful strategy for helping individuals who are trying to lose weight alter their eating and exercise habits. (Hollis et al., 2008) did a study on weight loss that included almost 1,700 people. The study found that those who wrote down what they ate every day lost twice as much weight as those who didn't. The research also showed that the best predictors of weight loss were how often people kept food diaries and how much they received support.

How to Make Food Journaling Work for You

Experts in the field of food journaling agree that accuracy and consistency are two of the most important parts of a good food diary. So, what should you jot down, you ask? The following items belong in any basic food journal:

- How much food do you consume? Make a record of how much food and drink you consume at each meal. Indicate the amount in ounces or ordinary household measures (cups, teaspoons, and tablespoons). It is advisable to measure and weigh your meals to the greatest extent possible. If you are away from home, attempt to approximate the portion as best you can.

- In what location are you eating? Write down every place you consume a meal, whether it's at home, in bed, in your car, on the sidewalk, at a friend's house, or at a restaurant. If you happen to be at a restaurant, for instance, note down the name of the place, what you ordered, and how much of the meal you consumed.

- What did you consume today? Write down everything you ate, how it was prepared (boiled, deep fried, baked, etc.), and what you drank throughout the day. Remember to include any extra toppings, sauces, condiments, or dressings such as sugar, butter, or tartar sauce.

- What time do you eat? Keeping track of the hours at which you consume food, might assist you in recognizing potentially problematic patterns, such as eating late at night. Keeping track of where you eat, what else you do when eating, and how you feel while eating may help you understand some of your routines and give more information.

- What emotions do you experience when eating? Are you happy, depressed, mad, nervous, lonely, bored, or stressed? By documenting how you feel at certain times, you may identify your triggers.

- With whom are you dining? If you aren't dining alone, who else may be present during your meal? A coworker, spouse, friend? Maybe you eat more when you're with certain people and don't even realize it.

- Do you have any other activities going on when you're eating? Are you interacting with friends or family, watching TV, using your laptop, or viewing something else? In this section, list any activities you do while eating or drinking. This may help you identify if you are a mindless eater and begin working on it.

How to Keep a Good Food Diary

- As soon as you finish the meal or drink, note it down. Avoid waiting until the end of the day since your memory will probably be less precise. Life gets hectic, and it is easy to forget the details if you wait until the end of the day. Therefore, writing it down immediately helps you get a more accurate picture of what you are really eating throughout the day or can help you plan ahead for what you are going to eat that day (which is even better.)

- Don't forget to mention any alcoholic drinks you take. Alcoholic beverages generally have a lot of sugar, so they can add up fast!

- You can help yourself further by using a smartphone app like Lose It! or MyFitnessPal. Calories and other dietary details are also available in these applications.

- When describing the meal or drink, be as descriptive as you can. Take an espresso as an example; when you drink this, pay close attention to the brand and the amount of your beverage. Similarly, after each meal, measure or estimate how much food you ate. Getting a measuring scale to help you weigh how much you're eating may help here.

So, You've Decided to Keep a Record of Everything You Eat. What Now?

Take a step back and review your entries after you've completed a week of food journaling. Look for any recurring tendencies, patterns, or routines; for instance, you may take into consideration items like:

- How nutritious is my diet? Pay close attention if you consume a lot of processed, sugary, or dairy-containing meals. Processed foods, in particular, include high proportions of added sugar, salt, and fat. Although these substances improve the flavor of the food we eat, consuming too much of them could result in major health problems, including obesity, heart disease, diabetes, and other cardiovascular diseases. Because of the extra sugar and fat, these foods also tend to have a higher calorie count. So, if you notice yourself nibbling on potato chips or buying a lot of ready-to-eat meals from the supermarket during the week, it's time to break the habit.

- Do I eat whole grains every day? The health benefits of whole grains are different from those of processed grains, which have been linked to problems like obesity and inflammation. A diet, high in whole grains, has been linked to several health benefits, such as a lower risk of diabetes, heart disease, and high blood pressure. Products created from whole grains are more satisfying than those made from refined grains, and some studies show that eating them may reduce the risk of obesity. A meta-analysis of 15 studies with almost 120,000 people found that eating the recommended three servings of whole grains every day was linked to a lower BMI and less belly fat (Harland & Garton, 2008).

- Do I eat or drink things that have sugar added to them? If yes, how often? The body may get its energy from sugar, a kind of carbohydrate. But long-term sugar consumption can cause weight gain. Sugar is in a lot of foods, both natural ones like fruit and processed ones like mass-produced bread and canned vegetables, not to mention sugary drinks and teas. For most adult women, the American Heart Association (AHA) recommends consuming no more than 100 calories per day (about 6 teaspoons or 24 grams of sugar), whereas, for most adult males, the recommended daily intake is 150 calories (around 9 teaspoons or 36 grams of sugar). Do my feelings have an impact on what I eat? When I'm worried or fatigued, do I find myself craving bad foods? Emotional eaters eat to get through difficult times. Emotional eating is a common phenomenon that affects a lot of people. Eating a bag of chips when sad or a chocolate bar after a challenging day at work are two examples of how it could manifest, but a person's life, health, happiness, and weight can all be hurt by emotional eating if it happens often or if it is the main way they deal with their feelings. When you give in to a yearning for food and eat it, your brain releases a neurotransmitter called dopamine, which makes you feel good. The process of craving something other than food and then fulfilling that craving will give your body the same chemical outcome. If you make a list of new habits to replace eating as a response to good or bad stress, you get the same "high" and a healthier outcome. I cannot create this list for you because you have to crave it. It needs to be something you enjoy that takes about the same amount of time as eating a snack, 2-5 minutes. When you retrain the habit of "stress eating" now, it will make keeping your weight off easier for life. Make this list today. Hand-write it. Put copies in your bathroom, on the refrigerator, in your purse or bag, and in your car. The next time you feel yourself starting to reach for food to cope, do something else on the list and note the feeling you have afterward. Accomplishment! Emotional eating can be caused by a lot of different things, not just bad emotions like stress.

People also say that they are triggered by boredom, exhaustion, social pressures, and unhealthy habits like rewarding themselves with sweet snacks all the time. Luckily, the first step in getting rid of emotional eating is to figure out what makes it happen in your life. Keeping a food journal might help you figure out the circumstances in which you are more prone to eat for emotional reasons than for physical ones.

You may learn more about your own eating patterns by monitoring this activity. How often do I eat while moving? When we're pressed for time, we turn to fast food, freezer meals, and even the closest gas station for quick, practical answers. Our bodies suffer as a result of the bad nourishment that results from this. Eating on the run also means we eat faster, which leads to us eating more. So, if you find that you tend to eat too much when you're in a hurry, work on stopping this habit. When we take the time to enjoy actual meals, our relationship with food changes. But of course, I do understand that life does get busy sometimes, so if you do fast food, almost every drive-through has a salad with grilled chicken, lettuce, and tomato. Gas stations have salads, fruit, or hard-boiled eggs available for quick protein. Don't let a busy schedule become an excuse for you to eat poorly. There are great choices out there. It's up to you to make the right choice in these moments to get the outcome you want-the healthiest you!

Craft Your Own Stylish Notebook

If you would rather not buy a ready-made diary, you can also make a personalized notebook in less than 15 minutes. You only need a few basic supplies and tools.

There are several ways to make notebooks, but this one has been the most reliable and flexible for my needs. In terms of page count and cover content, the sky's the limit (provided that you are able to make holes for the stitching in the cover). Don't overlook the importance of creating a stunning and unique design for the cover. If it looks attractive to your eyes, you will reach for it more often.

First Step—Compile all of your materials. You must first acquire a few tools and materials before you can begin. For equipment, you need a ruler, cutting board, needle, utility knife, sharpening steel, hammer, and leather punch. As for supplies, office paper; and the cover, cardboard, thread, paper, and tape (which is optional). Once you have the necessary equipment and materials, you may begin assembling it.

Second Step—First, Get several pieces of letter-size printer paper, cut them in half, and fold each piece in half. Once everything has been folded over, you will have a 4.25 x 5.5 inches notebook that fits perfectly in your pocket and that is large enough for both taking notes and drawing. Of course, there is no restriction on the size of the notebook; you may build it any way you choose.

Third Step—personalize the cover of your notebook with a sketch, print, or anything else you'd want to use before you sew it together. The possibilities here are almost endless.

Fourth Step—Make holes for sewing.

1. Arrange the pages facing the cover.

2. Mark the areas where the holes will be. Set the holes at a distance of 1 cm from the edge.

3. Use a punch to go through the holes. To do what you need to, you will essentially want a spike that can be struck with a hammer. Use anything that will create a circular hole as much as possible (this will eliminate tearing).

Fifth Step—Put It All Together: Start sewing on the inside of the notebook (at the bottom edge) and leave a short tail of thread to tie a knot at the beginning.

After stitching all the way through, go back to the beginning and tie a knot. Because of this, the binding between the pages and the cover is strong, solid, and long-lasting.

Sixth Step—Paper Tape (optional): You have the option of covering the notebook's spine with paper tape. Even though it's not necessary, this is a great way to finish off the design of a paper notebook.

Seventh Step—Trim the Extra Paper: Trim any extra paper that will protrude from the center of the notebook.

Eighth Step—If this notebook shouts "You!" when you look at it, you're finished. Everything can be altered to suit your preferences, including the size, number of pages, and layout. You will get a creative, practical, and very robust notebook using this technique. This makes for an aesthetically pleasing food journal. If you like the look and feel of it, you will be more likely to enjoy using it.

Measuring Food on the Fly

Portion sizes are important when trying to lose weight, and using a food scale or measuring cup will give you the most accurate results. Nevertheless, pulling out a food scale every time you sit down to eat may not always be a feasible option. So, you will have to make an educated guess about the right size of items sometimes. Fortunately, there are a few strategies you may use to accurately estimate portion sizes. Using your hands as a measuring tool is a quick and easy way to figure out how much food is in different serving sizes. Even if you're dining at a five-star establishment, the fact that it's a part of your body makes it a very practical measurement tool. However, since each person has somewhat different-sized hands, it's best to gain some experience with actual measurements before trying to guess how much something should be. When attempting to determine portion size, use these recommendations:

Protein consumption can be calculated using the palm of your hand. A serving of protein weighing 4 oz. is equal to one palm. Pork, poultry, beef, fish, and chicken are some examples of foods that you may measure a 4 oz. portion of.

A one-cup serving is roughly the size of a cupped hand. Food products like pasta, potatoes, almonds, and even ice cream can all be measured with the use of this tool.

A serving size of one tablespoon is about the same as the very tip of your thumb. Mayonnaise, cheese, salad dressings, creams, and peanut butter are all high in fat; hence, this instrument is used to determine how much of those foods a person consumes.

For measuring carbs, a fist works well. When trying to calculate how much rice, cereal, salad, fruit, or popcorn you've had, use this tool.

One teaspoon of oil or fat is about equal to the size of the thumbnail. Olive oil, butter, and salad dressings may all be measured with this.

Pre-planning and food preparation are keys to success in healthful eating. Sit down once a week when you have a small chunk of time. Look through your social calendar, the food in your fridge, freezer, and pantry, and plan your shopping list. Let the social calendar dictate which meals will be at home and which might be out. If those are home meals, plan the shopping list to use both what you have and buy only what you will need. If those meals will be fast food or restaurants, look at the menus online and determine what you will order. Pre-populate the food journal with your food plan for the week. Write meals in one color ink. For any changes that happen out of your control and do not end up going as planned, write in red. This makes for easy reference later. You can easily see what percentage of your food goes as planned and how many times you veered off the planned course.

The Power of a Good Attitude

I've already said that I'm a huge believer in positive thinking, and with good reason. Positive thinking and successful weight reduction go hand in hand, which shouldn't come as much of a surprise. I've found that keeping an optimistic frame of mind has helped me and my patients very much in our quest to shed pounds. I mean, just think about it, fixating on one's own past failure, and current discontentment makes weight loss difficult if not darn near impossible. And why is this the case? For the simple reason that dwelling on the bad causes us to give in to our desires, consume too much, and neglect our regular workout routine. Negative thinking patterns may hinder our weight reduction attempts in a number of ways, including beating ourselves up every time we consume the wrong foods, becoming preoccupied with what we can't eat, and approaching our workout routine with dread. A bad self-perception makes us feel helpless, unhappy, or uninspired, which increases the likelihood that we'll miss our daily exercise or eat a bag of chips to feel better. But understanding those emotions and changing those ideas into something more uplifting might really assist us in achieving our objectives. Here are some methods for developing a more optimistic outlook:

1. Keep cards with your objectives, motivational pictures, affirmations, and quotes visible.

    This keeps us motivated when we'd rather give up and serves as a helpful reminder to adopt an optimistic outlook. Imagine coming home from work absolutely exhausted and without any enthusiasm to exercise. However, seeing pictures of your goals plastered all over your wall would likely spur you on to go for that run won't it? Having something to look at that constantly reminds you that your dreams and goals are valuable is better than having nothing at all.

2. List Three Positive Aspects of Your Day

    These should be items over which you have some measure of influence, such as getting up early to jump some rope before even having breakfast, looking forward to a hot shower after a sweaty workout, or the taste of a chocolate protein shake for breakfast. See how your mood changes after a week of trying it out. The human brain has a natural inclination toward negativity, but this practice may help retrain it to see and appreciate the positive aspects of everyday life.

3. Stop Telling Yourself Bad Things

    If you find yourself having unproductive thoughts, consider replacing them with a string of positive affirmations. There are many books, podcasts, and videos online with endless positive affirmations.

Fact 3:

Macros Matter

Now that you have spent a week writing down and tracking everything as you eat it, and crafted a beautiful, aesthetically pleasing journal, you are ready to take food journaling to the next level. The term "macro" stands for macronutrients. Protein, carbohydrates, and fats are the three major classes of nutrients that make up the majority of the food that you consume and are the primary sources of the majority of the energy that you need. Keeping track of your macros means keeping track of how many grams of protein, carbohydrates, and fat you eat each day. You can make (or prepare to make) more informed, nutritious eating choices if you keep track of your macros.

The idea is similar to counting calories or points, but it goes further than that. Simply put, weight loss does not always occur when the calories burned exceed the calories consumed. Understanding the sources of those calories and how they affect your body is made easier with macro counting. Furthermore, it teaches you that not all calories are created equal. Let's suppose, for illustration purposes, that your daily calorie target is 2,000. Protein has a caloric value of four per gram. Therefore, a 125-gram serving of protein contains 500 calories, leaving 1,500 calories for fat and carbohydrates. Focusing more on the nutritional content of food is always preferable since it helps people pay closer attention to how their bodies are fueled and how their bodies respond. By concentrating on getting enough protein, and fats and paying more attention to the kind of carbs you are consuming rather than just calories alone, you may experience higher satiety (less hunger) and be better able to achieve your fitness goals. Another advantage of macro counting is that it is a versatile strategy. It's called "flexible dieting" because you still eat real food and don't starve your body. The phrase "If It Fits Your Macros," which means you may eat anything as long as it fits into your macros, is often used by those who track their percentage of carbohydrates/proteins/fats.

Should you now manipulate the system so you can consume just donuts? Obviously, no. But is it possible to occasionally indulge in a sweet treat or two and still achieve success? Yes! When you are counting macros, there is no such thing as a "cheat" meal; all that happens is that you have to rearrange some of your macros to make room for the new item. It is indeed possible to shed extra pounds, keep your muscles from wasting away, and keep your appetite in check by counting macros. Reading food labels and diet research out there can be really confusing, so paying attention to just these three categories can be really helpful. Some nutritionists worry that a macronutrient plan oversimplifies the problem and doesn't take into account the mental and social factors that lead to unhealthy eating. Still, some defend the simplicity as beneficial. I believe it is a great place to start. Take into account social/emotional issues as best you can with planning ahead, use the habit replacement tip mentioned earlier in this book, attend overeaters anonymous meetings if you need group support, reach out to mental health counselors when necessary, or you may reach me directly via www.lifelongmetaboliccenter.com if you need 1:1 help. Simplicity can be a beautiful thing, but please do not be too proud or scared to reach out when you need help. That's the blessing of the modern world and our abundant resources.

The Top 3 Best Ways to Use Macros to Lose Weight

Macros are totally conditional upon factors like age, height, and physicality. A person who leads a more sedentary lifestyle will need a lower total daily intake of carbohydrates and a higher total daily intake of protein than, say, an athlete would. For the most part, however, you can use these proportions as a general benchmark:

- If you workout for sixty minutes or less every day: 40% carbohydrates, 30% fat, and 30% protein

- With a daily workout regimen of one to two hours: 45% carbohydrates, 25% fat, and 30% protein

- If your everyday workout exceeds two hours, think about consulting Dr. Borre 1:1. To keep up that high physical output and healthily lose weight, you need customization.

Now that you know what the best macro ratio is, you can figure out how many macros you need and keep track of them in three easy steps:

1. Determine Your Caloric Requirements

   Again, the answer to this question exactly depends on things like your age, size, amount of exercise, and how much weight you want to lose, but a rough estimate would be to add one zero to your ideal body weight. For example: if you want to weigh 140 lbs., you should consume approximately 1400 calories per day.

2. Total the macros you used

   When you know how many calories you should consume each day, you can use your macronutrient ratio to calculate precisely how many grams of protein, fat, and carbohydrates to take in daily. A macro calculator, such as the one from freedieting.com, can help you save time because this requires a bit of calculating on your part. Using this technology, I found that a woman who ate 1,500 calories a day and worked out for 30 minutes most days of the week would need 150 grams of carbs, 112 grams of protein, and 50 grams of fat every day.

2. To Keep Tabs on Your Macros, Download an App Like MyfitnessPal or Use One of Your Beautifully Crafted Journals

   You should keep note of the quantities of each macronutrient that you consume at each meal and snack now that you know how much you require. Using a meal tracker app is one efficient method for doing this. Using these numbers, you can pre-plan your week, prep foods ahead of time, and then just work the plan! If the concept of a macro diet as a whole, leaves you feeling overwhelmed, just know that you are not alone in this feeling. There is no doubt that dedication is necessary for this level of meticulous tracking. I understand that it can be especially difficult if you're someone who dines out often. Therefore, I'm suggesting a simpler, but less accurate, way, which is to simply use your eyes. Make a bit more than a quarter of your plate lean protein and around a quarter of your plate whole grains or starchy veggies (like baked potatoes) if you're trying to get your macros in but detest monitoring meals or can't at the moment. You should fill up the rest of your plate with vegetables that don't have starch but are still counted as carbohydrates. You don't have to worry about including fat on your plate if you include foods like salad greens dressed in a vinaigrette or chicken grilled in olive oil that already contains fat. And if it doesn't satisfy your hunger, load up on the green stuff. You won't be able to verify that your macros are in the perfect 30/30/40 range with this strategy, but you will be able to make sure you eat enough protein and avoid consuming too many refined carbohydrates. Also, it will aid you in controlling your portion sizes. In fact, doing both can speed up your progress toward a slimmer physique.

Pay Attention to Your Carb Intake

What would you say if I asked you whether or not you eat a balanced, nutritious diet? Well, assuming you're like the majority of Americans, you'd likely respond, "Heck yes." Approximately 75% of Americans say they don't worry about what they consume because they believe they eat relatively healthily. But this is simply untrue. In fact, according to (Paddock, 2015), a shocking 76% of Americans weren't getting enough fruit, and 87% weren't getting enough vegetables. The fact that the average size of our portions is only becoming larger really isn't helping our obesity problem. As it stands, the percentage of obese people in the United States is now more than 25% in 48 states, 35% in nine states, and 30% in 31 states.

In fact, an investigation of dietary patterns by (Shan et al., 2019) found that Americans consume much more saturated fat and refined carbs than is healthy. The study, which followed 43,996 people from 1999 to 2016, revealed that Americans had gradually reduced their use of "low-quality" carbohydrates, including overly processed grains and sugary snack items. But in absolute terms, the decline is merely 3%. Even so, Americans still don't eat enough of the healthier types of carbs. Whole grains high in fiber, fruits, and vegetables are examples of high-quality carbohydrates. Low-quality carbohydrates make up 42% of the average American diet, whereas high-quality carbs make up just 9%. Not only will these poor carbohydrates likely exacerbate your weight loss troubles, but they may also significantly raise your risk of type 2 diabetes and cardiovascular disease. Especially as we age, our vulnerability to these sorts of things increases. So, don't just think of clean eating as a good way to keep weight off. The wellness of your body depends on it as well.

In contrast to whole grains, processed carbohydrates have all their fiber, vitamins, and minerals removed, making them immediately absorbed by the body upon consumption. Our body's ability to burn fat is abruptly overridden by this, which also causes a sharp rise in blood sugar and the production of large amounts of insulin. Because of this, our body does not utilize the processed carbohydrates we ate as fuel and instead stores them as extra body fat. Having said that, eliminating all carbohydrates from your diet is not always the best course of action, so remember everything is in moderation.

While eliminating ALL carbs may be fruitful for a select few, most people would find it unsatisfying and unsustainable. That is why, after you assess your food diary and understand your daily eating patterns if you are overeating carbs, you need to make a personalized plan on how to gradually reduce your carb intake for your desired goal. If you notice you eat a lot of processed carbs throughout the day like white bread, pasta, white flour, donuts, etc., you should make an active attempt to replace them with higher-quality carbs. If say, for example, you notice from your notebook that you have a tendency to eat a lot of cupcakes when you are watching TV. Well now begin to implement steps to change this habit. You can begin by replacing all those sweet desserts with naturally sweet fruit like apricots or apples. So now every time you find yourself mindlessly eating away at least it'll be fiber-filled goodies. By the end of your show, you'll probably find that you ate less food than usual too. That's better for most because cutting out carbs entirely is unsustainable in the long term.

I see a lot of patients in my clinic who were successful at cutting carbs, but the minute they came back, so did the weight-and it brought friends. Fiber's presence in food can slow digestion in the stomach, helping you feel fuller for longer. Also, high-fiber foods are low in calories, which makes for a good strategy. Want the best news ever? You can actually eat carbs every day without having to worry about getting fat. People mistake all carbohydrates as being the same and having the same effect on the body. It's actually complex carbs that support our ideal well-being, while simple processed carbohydrates are what essentially causes weight gain. Simple carbs have the same addictive qualities as sugar and therefore are also easy to grow hooked on.

The brain's reward circuitry is profoundly affected by them. Dopamine, which is responsible for emotions like pleasure and reward, is released when we eat carbohydrates. When you eat processed carbohydrates, your brain responds by generating a lot of dopamine almost instantaneously. This feel-good moment is what makes people want to continue eating. If ingested to an excessive degree and on a frequent basis, this will cause the brain to get used to it, at which point it will "require" simple carbohydrates in order to feel satisfied. And so starts the addictive loop. That explains in part why so many Americans consume so many processed foods without giving them a second thought.

As I indicated before, the answer isn't to eliminate all carbohydrates; rather, it's to swap them out for more complex ones and usually reduce the amount. Complex carbohydrates are digested quite differently from simple carbs, despite the fact that they also convert to sugar in the body. Due to their high fiber, vitamin, and mineral content, which enters the system more gradually, complex carbohydrates help slow down digestion and maintain healthy blood sugar levels. After incorporating them into your regular diet, you won't feel dependent on unhealthy foods anymore since it doesn't significantly raise your blood sugar, release high quantities of the hormone that stores fat in your body, or secrete dopamine in the brain. Examples of processed carbohydrates are anything that has been man-made like cereal, tortillas, bread, or pasta. Simple carbohydrates are those that come from the earth like rice, potatoes, yams, couscous, or zucchini.

What Is a Micronutrient?

While the phrase "macronutrients" refers to proteins, lipids, and carbs, the term "micronutrients" refers to vitamins and minerals. Generally speaking, your body cannot create vitamins and minerals; thus, humans must get their micronutrients from the diet. They are also known as vital nutrients because of this. Vitamins are created by plants and animals and are susceptible to decomposition when exposed to high temperatures, acids, or air. Contrarily, minerals are inorganic, found in either soil or water, and are not decomposable under normal conditions. Whenever you eat, you take in the minerals and vitamins that the food you ate originally had.

To ensure that you are getting adequate vitamins and minerals, it is better to consume a range of meals since each item has varied amounts of micronutrients. Since each vitamin and mineral has a distinct purpose in your body, an appropriate intake of all micronutrients is essential for achieving maximum health. Vitamins and minerals are necessary for normal development, immune system function, brain maturation, and many other vital activities. Some micronutrients, depending on how they are used, can also aid in the prevention and treatment of certain illnesses. One potential reason for weight gain is micronutrient insufficiency. A balanced diet is SO important for good health, and that includes both Macro and Micronutrients in sufficient quantities. Four hot ones right now are:

Calcium

Although best known for strengthening bones and teeth, calcium also aids in maintaining a healthy weight. There are studies out there that demonstrate calcium consumption can truly help you lose weight, so do not cut these out entirely. Moderation again is key. I have personally seen these results with my own patients. It's important to note that when you cut down on your calorie intake generally, meals high in calcium are proven to help you lose weight.

Potassium

Potassium, a little-spoken-of micronutrient, is a vitamin that is helpful for weight reduction and is essential for helping muscles recover after exercise. Additionally, it aids in the body's detoxification process and may lessen bloating by eliminating too much salt. Both the heart and the kidneys benefit from potassium's presence. Bananas, mushrooms, spinach, and sweet potatoes, are all good sources of potassium.

Fats in omega-3

Two health advantages of eating foods high in omega-3 fatty acids are a healthier heart and skin. As an added bonus, it may help you lose weight by making you feel fuller for longer. Metabolic rate and the number of calories burned during exercise may both increase from supplementation with omega-3 fatty acids. Walnuts, soybeans, canola oil, chia seeds, and fatty fish like salmon, sardines, and tuna are examples of foods high in omega-3 fatty acids.

Magnesium

With the help of this micronutrient, bloating, and water retention can be minimized, and blood flow enhanced. In those who are overweight or obese, magnesium may control insulin levels and, therefore, blood sugar levels. The mineral magnesium may be found in abundance in foods like beans, nuts, and seeds, as well as in green, leafy vegetables.

Shelly's Story-When Keto Isn't All Bad

After being told that he had cancer, my friend Jeff, husband and father of three boys, chose to follow the ketogenic diet over chemotherapy and conventional methods of treatment. The popularity of the keto diet is unprecedented. The keto diet is so popular that many dieters credit it for their success in losing weight-plus the fact that it is extensively promoted by so many celebrities and fitness "gurus" on Instagram.

Shelly, his wife, decided she would do it with him along with their whole family. They had MAJOR motivation to follow it to the letter and long term. He was given a short prognosis for life expectancy. Jeff believes that despite doctors saying his tumor was incurable, it shrank as a result of his diet, which comprises very little to no carbs. Almost no surgeon would even consider operating on it. After a period of time, one surgeon was able to successfully remove a portion of it. When you have cancer, diagnostic testing utilizes sugar for imaging because it goes directly to "feed" cancer, therefore making it easy to visualize. Doesn't it make sense that we wouldn't want to feed cancer? Shelly lost weight and felt amazing. Jeff went on to be the longest-living person on record at the time of his type of cancer. Although a few studies have shown it could be able to treat specific cancers, the diet is not one that is often advised by doctors for the prevention or treatment of cancer, and I'm not sure why, so talk to your doctor if this is a concern for you or a family member. Another potential reason why the diet may help treat tumors is that it has the potential to inhibit tumor development, safeguard healthy cells, reduce inflammation, and enhance the efficacy of anti-cancer medications. Use common sense, consult your doctor, and make educated decisions based on what makes the most sense for you, but overall, very low-carb diets are tough to sustain unless you are highly motivated to do it forever.

There are a lot of articles about the diet online, and stores carry a wide range of foods that are good for people who are on it. Even many of my own patients want to give it a try and often ask me how to get started. The ketogenic diet, or "keto" for short, entails eating very little carbohydrates and a high-fat diet. When you eat a low-carbohydrate ketogenic diet, your body quickly burns up the carbs stored in your muscles and liver as glycogen. You switch to burning fat after your glycogen reserves are exhausted. During this phase, many individuals see significant weight reduction, which is why so many other people are eager to give it a try.

Why to NOT Keto

However, despite these assertions and interests, the majority of health care providers, including physicians and nutritionists, do not advocate for it. The ketogenic diet is not something I recommend to my patients since I am not a fan of it myself. First of all, it's not a healthy approach to maintain weight loss, and I know this from personal experience since practically every patient I've treated who had been on the keto diet gained the weight back as soon as they quit the diet. This was the case with American actress, producer, and fitness expert Tamra Judge. The Glendale, California-born reality personality has a history of experimenting with new diets and exercise routines, and in June 2021 she stated that she would be trying the ketogenic diet (Berg, 2021). Although Tamara is renowned for her diet-related open-mindedness, she wasn't a fan of the keto diet before attempting it because of all the health risks, but she gave it a try nonetheless in the hopes that it might help with her autoimmune difficulties.

A couple of months after beginning the diet, one of her Instagram followers asked whether she was still following the low-carb plan; she responded, "No, I put on weight while on Keto," with a sad emoji. Nutritionists aren't fans for a variety of reasons, not only long-term maintenance. The lack of fruits and whole grains on the ketogenic diet makes me dislike it even more since I know that it might induce constipation in certain people. Constipation is a miserable condition in and of itself, but anybody who has suffered from it knows that if it persists for an extended period of time, it may also cause hemorrhoids and rectal tears. Plus, while you're out and about with the family and kids, the last thing you want to do is spend a long time in the restroom because of constipation. On the ketogenic diet, you can't eat a lot of starchy vegetables, lentils, or yogurt. This makes you more likely to be malnourished. It may also raise your risk of heart disease due to its high saturated fat content. The keto diet's exclusion of whole foods groups long term is a big turn-off for my scientific brain. The rigor of the diet is a problem as well. It's very difficult for a single person to follow a lifestyle that calls for so many sacrifices, such as calculating carbs, cutting out whole food categories, monitoring protein consumption, and limiting food options within authorized groups., but to keep these limitations in place over time is extremely unlikely for anybody. Parents who are attempting to set a positive example for their children in regard to diet and nutrition want to follow guidelines that appear healthy and well-balanced.

How to NOT Keto

As you may have gathered from my above text, I am not a proponent of the keto diet. I have seen far too many patients come to me after doing it short term only to have acquired more weight in a short time afterward. That being said, I do believe there is oodles of research out there about the typical American diet and culturally how excessive our "normal" carb intake is. So even though I won't tell you to go "no carb" or "low carb", what you may need is likely less than you think is normal now. For exact numbers on macro counts for your body, you may contact me directly at www.lifelongmetaboliccenter.com.

How to Exercise After 40 to Lose Fat and Gain Muscle

No matter what program you choose, the six things below should be the most important parts of your workout routine if you want to gain lean muscle mass, become more physically active, and look better after 40.

Always Warm Up

The warm-up phase of our exercise regimen becomes more crucial as we age. The last thing you want is to be hurt and unable to get in your weekly workouts, play with your children, or go to work. Also, as we get older, our bodies tend to lose some of their flexibility. Therefore, warming up is essential if you want to continue exercising regularly in the future, and it's also crucial to prevent injuries. Warm up thoroughly, and pay specific attention to your shoulders, hips, ankles, and knees. A nice place to start is with some dynamic stretches and a little mild cardio. Just always keep in mind that you're trying to prevent injuries because they can really hold you back from attaining your goals. It may take more time than in the past to bounce back from a setback as well, so it's best to avoid them if possible.

Weekly Weight Lifting

It's possible that you won't be able to lift weights four times a week like you used to. Perhaps due to time or perhaps body restrictions. Yet, if you want to gain muscle, lifting is a great way to trigger the growth response necessary. Exercises that train many muscle groups and joints at once, such as squats, deadlifts, bench presses, and cleans, are the greatest for increasing strength. Lifting two or three times per week, 3 sets, with around 8–15 repetitions per set, is a tried-and-true strength training regimen for gaining muscle beyond 40. (Warmup sets are recommended before attempting these.) To maximize improvement, keep your routine simple and make little weight increases per week. But if you're a beginner, you should definitely start with lower weights to avoid injury. You may get discomfort in some body parts, such as the wrists, elbows, and so on, but you should not have PAIN. You can lift more weight by using complex movements in combination with these rep schemes, which will result in a bigger metabolic reaction.

Workout With Cardio Several Times Each Week

Weightlifting is fantastic, but for optimal results, you must also do some cardiovascular exercise. When we do 30–40 minutes of cardiovascular activity, it helps to boost our metabolism for the next 24 hours. In addition to jogging (or fast walking if you're new to it), jumping rope, swimming, burpees, squat jumps, and cycling, you might also practice other exercises that you find enjoyable that raise your heart rate and break a sweat.

Rest, Rest, Rest

If you want to gain muscle beyond the age of 40, sleep is a necessity. The body overflows with feel-good chemicals that encourage recuperation and repair when we are sleeping. (Not just skeletal muscles, but also the nervous system and internal organs.) If you aren't getting enough shut-eye, it may be one of the factors adding to your weight gain. Getting a good night's sleep is another way to boost your strength at the gym. Your exercise routine can deteriorate if you don't receive enough of it. As you get older, you may find it harder to get enough sleep due to work, children, and other factors in your life. But it should be one of your top concerns if you don't want to gain weight or do want to keep your muscles from getting smaller. And by that, I don't simply mean getting more sleep but also making sure that the sleep you do receive is good sleep. Sleep in a dark room, consistently as opposed to broken sleep/naps, no tech before bed. These can all increase the quality of your sleep.

Power Proteins

Protein is the nutritional building block for growing lean muscle. After 40, protein needs to be given even more attention than in our younger days. When you are between the ages of 40 and 50, your protein demands rise to roughly 1-1.2 grams per kilogram, or 75–90 grams per day for a 75-kilogram individual (Wempen, 2022). Regular exercisers also have greater requirements, ranging from 1.1 to 1.5 grams per kilogram. 1.2–1.7 grams per kilogram are required for those who routinely lift weights or are preparing for a race.

Get Your Supplements

Some supplements can be really helpful in your muscle-gaining mission. Though do Understand that supplements are just the "extra 10%" that get you where you need to go. They don't take the place of a disciplined workout regimen or a healthy diet. To assist you in muscle building, consider the following:

- Fish oil may help you exercise and lift more frequently by lowering inflammation.

- Whey protein: Nutritional supplementation with whey protein powder after exercise has been shown to hasten recovery. Protein shakes like Quest, or Fairlife Elite can be easy, portable ways to get more delicious protein in your life.

- BCAA's-Branch Chain Amino Acids are a great way to hasten muscle recovery after your workout. Most have great fruity flavors and feel very much like a post-workout treat.

Myths Surrounding the Keto Diet

Myth #1: When on keto, you are continually burning fat

So, you already know that the key "benefit" of the ketogenic diet is that it puts your body into a state known as "fat-burning mode." You've switched from using sugar as an energy source to using fat as fuel 24/7. And to be fair, this is correct. Ketosis refers to the condition in which your body begins to burn fat. That being said, even if your body is in ketosis, you primarily burn food fat before any stored body fat. Always being in a state of ketosis does not guarantee weight loss. To ensure success, you still have to be in a calorie deficit, stay there for an extended period of time, and not break your fast with garbage food.

Myth #2: When Eating Keto, You Don't Need to Track Your Calories.

Some advocates of the ketogenic diet claim that, once in ketosis, calories no longer count and that you may eat as much butter and bacon as you want without gaining weight. This is such an annoying myth for me, especially when you think about how important the quality of foods is whether or not you're trying to lose weight. Calorie deficit is easy to understand. You burn off a certain amount of calories each day. If you eat more calories than you exert, you will gain weight. And you'll lose weight if you consume fewer calories than you expend. Simple as that. Pair this with eating the right ratio of carb/fat/protein per day, and you've got a winner. You can't tell me eating bacon and butter in excess truly makes sense for good health, right?

Myth #3: Everyone Has Equal Carbohydrate Needs

Your own body will determine how many carbs you should consume-not a generic restriction number and definitely not ZERO. When first beginning a ketogenic or other extremely low-carb diets, it is easy to underestimate the extent to which your diet will restrict carbohydrate intake. Well, in order to assist the body in entering ketosis, followers often start on the lower end of the 20–50 gram range of carbs per day. But of course, with some tweaks (such as increasing your exercise), you may be able to push intake further. Those who have trouble using fat as fuel due to genetics may find it very challenging, if not impossible to lose weight by using this dieting method.

Myth #4: There's No Such Thing as Too Much Protein

Although low in carbohydrates, it is not the same as the Atkins Diet. A breakfast of eggs and smoked salmon and a supper of steak may seem delicious, but protein should be consumed in proportion with other nutrients. This is one distinction between the ketogenic and the Atkins diets. Any more protein than your body needs may be turned into glucose, which can cause a spike in blood sugar. Furthermore, a keto dieter who already has high amounts of ketones in their body may have problems due to the breakdown of amino acids in the protein, which may result in an increase in ketones.

Myth #5: The Keto Diet Is the Most Effective Weight Loss Strategy

In case you hadn't heard, there isn't a "magic bullet" diet that works for everyone. Keto is not always the perfect diet for you just because your buddy lost weight on it, or it seems like everyone is talking about it. The most common misconception I see in my line of work these days is that the ketogenic diet is the holy grail of weight loss. The truth is that while it's tempting to try the latest fad diet, the key to long-term success is settling on a healthy eating pattern that you can stick to AND having an answer to two questions. What measures will I take to LOSE weight? What am I going to do to MAINTAIN the weight loss life-long? Those should be two different answers as you don't want to LIVE on a diet.

Fat Is Not the Enemy

Repeat after me "The only thing that is really bad for me is eating too much saturated fat and trans fat from processed foods." I know it's popular to hate fat and think that there are no healthy kinds, but this is very false! Take the creamy, deliciousness of avocado as an example. It is rich in beneficial fats that support our body's ability to absorb nutrients, produce hormones, protect organs, produce energy, develop cells, and insulate against cold.

However, if you're not an avocado fan and aren't sure how to tell healthy fats from harmful ones, you're not alone in your bafflement.

Here, I've sifted through the nonsense to tell you which fats will help you achieve your objectives and which ones you should stay away from. Let's start off by discussing healthy fats. The body benefits particularly from the naturally occurring fats found in whole foods. Fats are the last to exit the digestive system, making them the most satisfying since they are both satiating and a source of energy. As a result, fats, particularly those made from real fats, can help us feel filled for longer and prevent us from overeating. What kinds of fats are thus worth watching out for? Well, to begin with, unsaturated fat is the nutritional facts' golden child.

In terms of health advantages, this kind of fat gets an A+. It falls into two groups: monounsaturated fats (MUFAs) and polyunsaturated fats (PUFAs). PUFAs have been shown to raise good cholesterol levels while simultaneously lowering LDL cholesterol levels (HDL). Plus, the risk of developing heart disease is decreased by the consumption of PUFAs. That is three big wins already! The omega-3 and omega-6 fatty acids that are good for the heart may be found in PUFAs. Hello, beautiful skin and lustrous hair, as well as a plethora of other health advantages! While keeping HDL levels the same, MUFAs may lower LDL. Moreover, several studies suggest they may lessen the dangers of cardiovascular disease. Over the years, you've probably heard that saturated fat raises Cholesterol levels, making it a bad food choice. However, recent research indicates that consuming more saturated fat is also linked to an increase in HDL, which lowers overall cholesterol levels.

At the moment, fewer than 10% of our daily calories should come from saturated fat, according to Health and Human Services (HHS) and the U.S. Department of Agriculture (USDA). Researchers, however, are advocating for revisions to this guideline since replacing our preferred lipids with processed carbohydrates may have unintended negative consequences. In fact, a meta-analysis led by (Dehghan et al., 2017) found that replacing saturated fat with refined carbohydrates like white rice and bread may raise the risk of cardiovascular disease. On the other hand, consuming more fat overall (both saturated and unsaturated) was linked to a reduced risk. The key is moderation; eating healthy doesn't require that you wrap every meal in bacon, but it also doesn't need you to avoid that whole-milk cappuccino. (You should cut down on the bread and butter and try to avoid eating too many refined carbohydrates and saturated fats at once.) What makes fat saturated? At room temperature, test the consistency. When left at room temperature, saturated fats remain solid whereas unsaturated fats remain liquid. Taking a look at the processing and packaging of the fat is a good way to get a sense of which fats are good for you. Bad fats are more likely to be present in prepackaged, processed meals. Good fats are more likely to be found in whole, unprocessed foods. Therefore, some saturated fats to consider eating are things like full-fat dairy products like butter, cheese, and cream, lard, and solid oils like palm, kernel, and coconut. True, our bodies need fat to function properly, but not all fats are the same. Fats are a great source of energy, and as long as we stay away from the unnatural trans fats found in fried meals and pastries, we should be good to go.

However, it's also OK and sometimes even advantageous to eat naturally occurring trans fats, such as those present in various meat and dairy products. Humans have been consuming these natural trans fats for ages after all, unlike synthetic trans fats. Therefore, as we've seen, fat can be a healthy element of your plan whether you're aiming to lose weight or maintain your present weight on the scale. However, this does not imply that you should rely only on fats for ALL of your nutritional needs. Because fat has a higher proportion of calories per gram than other macronutrients, eating too much of it may contribute to weight gain. Each gram of fat contains about 9 calories. The calorie content of both protein and carbohydrates is four. For the body to be well nourished, the diet must be balanced and include high-quality fats.

Fact 4:

Control Constipation—You Won't See This in the Books for Youngins

If you have ever suffered from constipation, you know how awful it can be. Constipation is one of the most frequent Gastrointestinal issues among US adults. Every year, at least 2.5 million individuals seek medical attention for constipation. Less than three bowel motions per week or stool movements that are difficult to pass are signs of constipation. This may lead to extra unnecessary time spent using the toilet and straining. Constipation is often seen as a symptom of an underlying illness, rather than a disease since its causes differ. Constipation may have many causes, but dehydration and a lack of fiber in the diet are the two common ones.

Constipation may also be brought on by stress, hormonal changes, spinal injuries, muscular issues, malignancies, and structural issues with the digestive system, among other, more severe conditions. The range of the total gut transit is about between 10 and 73 hours. However, the number of bowel movements you have in a given day is impacted by a variety of factors, including your age, gender, eating and exercise routines, as well as your current state of health. Although three or fewer times per week may be detrimental, there is no suggested minimum number of bowel movements. People over 50 and women are more likely to have constipation. This is especially true for the elderly, who, in comparison to their younger selves, are less likely to engage in physical activity, have slower metabolisms, and have weaker muscular contractions all throughout their digestive tract. The use of some drugs by older individuals, particularly when their health isn't being taken care of, tends to make them constipated. And when it comes to women, those who are pregnant are the ones who are most likely to be affected by it.

Pregnant women are more prone to constipation due to changes in their hormones. Because the growing baby puts pressure on the bowels, they move more slowly during pregnancy and sometimes even after. Not being able to poop doesn't mean you stop craving food, and this can easily result in weight gain. This uncomfortable feeling of not being able to poop when you really want leads many to turn to laxatives. People use laxatives, which are drugs, to assist in accelerating bowel movements or to loosen up a stool in order to make passing easier. Additionally, they are becoming a well-liked weight reduction technique. There is a widespread belief that using laxatives may facilitate an increased frequency of bowel movements, which in turn can make weight reduction more rapid, straightforward, and uncomplicated. And while laxatives have been shown to hasten weight reduction, this effect is only short-lived. Many different forms of laxatives achieve their desired effects by drawing water from the body into the intestines. This enables the stool to absorb more water and move more smoothly through the digestive tract. The only weight you will lose with this strategy is the water you pass via your bowels. The idea that laxatives are a useful tool for managing weight lacks any strong supporting data for long-term use. You don't necessarily need drugs to cure your constipation unless it's chronic, then in that case I would advise consulting your doctor. If not, though, there are still other better and healthier alternatives to treating constipation, which I go into depth about below.

Consider Magnesium Citrate

Magnesium Citrate is an all-natural supplement used to help bowel movements. It effectively binds the food in your gut to help carry it along the way at a reasonable rate. Typically, this is the job done by carbohydrates. If you are on a reduced carbohydrate diet, you may then need to supplement with Magnesium Citrate to temporarily take over this job. Brief bouts of constipation may be alleviated with the use of magnesium citrate. When you go to the bathroom more often, your stool gets softer and easier to pass. Magnesium citrate is a widely used, straightforward treatment for sporadic constipation when administered as directed. And for people with no health concerns, magnesium citrate is typically safe. Therefore, unless you consume too much of it, it shouldn't create urgency or sudden visits to the toilet. You don't need a prescription to get it, and you can find it at most stores like Walmart or Target although amazon has the best versions I have found.

Water, as noted in Fact number one, is very vital and possibly the greatest drink for helping with constipation relief. Drinking more water makes the most sense since chronic dehydration can lead to constipation. Water not only keeps you hydrated, but it also stimulates digestion. Some persons who suffer from chronic idiopathic constipation or indigestion (also known as dyspepsia) believe that sparkling water is even more beneficial than regular tap water in easing their symptoms. However, fizzy drinks like sugary soda should be avoided since they might have negative health impacts and may exacerbate constipation. Magnesium citrate in greater dosages is often prescribed by doctors as a colon cleanse prior to surgery. If someone consumes too much of the substance, it may have a strong impact. If you decide to use magnesium citrate, be sure to follow all dosing and storage directions provided by the manufacturer. Magnesium Citrate tablets are best with zero additives if possible. Avoid gel caps or liquids as they may have added unnecessary ingredients. Take it at bedtime.

Who Ought to Stay Away From Magnesium Citrate?

Most individuals can safely take magnesium citrate in the right amounts; however, there are certain people who should not. If you have a renal illness, nausea, stomach discomfort, vomiting, a sudden change in your bowel habits that has lasted more than a week, or if you are on a low-sodium or restricted-sodium diet, see your doctor before taking any magnesium citrate. Some drugs may be less effective when used with magnesium citrate because it might reduce their absorption. For instance, magnesium citrate may prevent some HIV medicines from functioning effectively if you are taking them. Therefore, find out from your doctor if any supplements or prescriptions you are taking might be affected by magnesium citrate. If you're experiencing rectal bleeding, then you shouldn't be using magnesium citrate. It should also be avoided by those who have had certain surgeries or have particular medical conditions. Magnesium citrate should not be used by anybody who often has prolonged bouts of constipation. Only mild or infrequent instances of constipation can be safely treated with magnesium. It is not meant for continued usage. The reason is that the body might develop a tolerance to magnesium citrate, making it difficult to defecate without the use of laxatives, if it is used on a frequent basis. To discover long-term treatments for their symptoms, anybody with persistent constipation should speak with their doctor.

Another Reason Why You Should Get All of Your Steps In

It's natural to want to curl up in the fetal position and hold your stomach when constipation strikes, but getting up off your bed and moving about will benefit you a great deal more. Physical exercise is perhaps one of the best lifestyle tricks for maintaining regularity and relaxing your bowels. It encourages the muscles in the gut wall to spontaneously contract by including frequent moderate-to-vigorous exercise in your daily routine. Jogging, water aerobics, and yoga are all examples of physical exercise, but even brisk walking can help with constipation difficulties. To successfully acquire fitness and good health, walk at a speed that is dictated by your metabolic rate. If you're told to walk at a brisk pace, all that implies is that you should walk a little quicker than usual. Your fitness level has a significant role in determining your pace. 100 steps per minute, or 3 to 3.5 miles per hour, is what most fitness professionals define as a brisk walking speed. Therefore, a great method to boost your physical activity is to go on brisk walks, which are considered moderate-intensity exercise. This kind of physical activity increases your heart rate, causes you to breathe more rapidly, and promotes good cardiovascular health. (Tantawy et al., 2017) examined middle-aged obese women who had persistent constipation for a period of 12 weeks. When compared to the control group that did not engage in any physical exercise, the first group's constipation symptoms and quality of life scores improved more after three weeks of walking on a treadmill for 60 minutes each time. Constipation is also related to an unbalanced gut bacterial population.

(Morita et al., 2019) conducted a research study in which they compared the makeup of gut microbes in the two groups to examine the impact of fast walking vs workouts that developed trunk muscles (such as planks). The research showed that aerobic exercises like brisk walking can increase the amount of Bacteroides in the gut, which are an important part of good gut bacteria. Studies have shown that people feel better when they walk quickly for at least 20 minutes every day, most days of the week. Recommendations for how long people should walk at a brisk pace differ.

What to do first

It's still crucial to consult your healthcare practitioner before beginning any walking program, even when walking may be exactly what you need at the moment. If you take any drugs or have any medical issues, then seeing a doctor is even more crucial. Some examples of this include experiencing lightheadedness, faintness, or difficulty breathing when on foot. If you take any drugs or have any medical issues, then seeing a doctor prior to beginning a vigorous exercise plan is recommended. To avoid hurting yourself, remember to never ignore your body's cues and do so much that you risk injury. To help you remain focused, look for a walking buddy who is also willing to serve as your accountability partner. Think about giving yourself non-food rewards when you achieve your objectives. This will make you feel proud, and you'll most likely want to continue. To track your daily speed and steps, you can use an app or a speedometer. Another option is to investigate if there are any walking groups in your area. Working out with other people is always more fun, plus you end up doing more workouts. Make the commitment to begin walking your way to improved health right now, no matter how you choose to go about it.

Why Leafy Green Vegetables Are Great

In some situations, the simplest of explanations will do the trick. Making a big salad with spinach and other leafy greens can help with constipation. This is because they hold a lot of insoluble fiber which has also been shown to reduce IBS symptoms. Insoluble fiber levels are often high in vegetables and certain fruits. Insoluble fiber doesn't break down in water or digestive fluids, so it mostly stays the same as it moves through the digestive system. Insoluble fiber is not a source of calories since it is not at all digested, but on the other hand, when soluble fiber reaches the stomach and intestines, it dissolves in water and digestive juices. The bacteria in the large intestine then break it down into a gel-like material, releasing gasses and a few calories in the process.

Consuming a lot of insoluble fiber while your stomach is inflamed is similar to rubbing a wire brush against an open cut, even though soluble fiber may be relaxing for the gut. That hurts, and it's not fun. If you like kale, arugula, and spinach in your salads rather than iceberg lettuce, give it a try. However, in addition to being high in fiber, green vegetables like spinach, broccoli, and Brussels sprouts are also excellent providers of vitamins C and K as well as folate. Stools made with these greens are heavier and have more mass, making it simpler for the intestines to move them along. Cooked spinach provides 4.7 grams of fiber, or 19% of the RDI, per cup (180 grams). If you want to increase the amount of spinach in your diet, you may make a pie, quiche, or soup using spinach as the main ingredient.

To increase the fiber content of salads or sandwiches, raw baby spinach or delicate greens may be used. Also, Brussels sprouts are very healthy. Just five sprouts give you 14% of your daily fiber needs and only 41 calories. They taste great hot or cold, and you can cook them by boiling, steaming, grilling, or roasting, and a single cup of broccoli has 2.4 grams of fiber (91 grams). This is 10% of the recommended daily intake of fiber. It's versatile enough to be used in both hot and cold dishes, from salads to stews to raw additions to hot soups. Because it can't be digested, insoluble fiber helps prevent constipation by sticking to other parts of the digestive process that are getting ready to form stool and by soaking up liquids while it rests in the digestive system. Its presence speeds up the movement and digestion of waste, which lowers the risk of constipation and GI blockage.

Smooth Moves Tea

The natural laxative known as Smooth Move tea is a combination of organic herbs that is sold as a tea. It is supposed to help cure constipation in as little as six to twelve hours after taking it. The main ingredient is senna, a strong plant that grows in Africa and India. It is a well-liked component of constipation cure medicines due to its natural laxative effects. The active ingredient in senna, called sennoside, causes your bowels to contract and helps increase the amount of water and electrolytes in your colon, both of which help you go to the bathroom. Licorice, bitter fennel, cinnamon, ginger, coriander, and sweet orange are other components in Smooth Move tea. These herbs are designed to ease gastrointestinal discomfort and lessen cramping. Smooth Move tea preparation calls for 8 ounces (240 ml) of boiling water to be poured over a tea bag, followed by 10-15 minutes of steeping time with the lid on the mug. Teas that make you poop, like Smooth Move, are sometimes used to help people lose weight. This kind of tea causes bowel movements and hinders the body's ability to absorb water from your colon again. So, it may help you go to the bathroom and make you lose fluids, which can both help reduce bloating and give you a sense of lightness. Smooth Move tea's principal component is senna, a natural laxative that has been used for hundreds of years. It causes bowel movements to be more frequent, heavier, and softer. Smooth Move tea may also help keep you from getting hemorrhoids because it makes going to the bathroom easier.

Fact 5:

Everyone Exercise

We have already covered Macros and the importance of the right balance of certain foods and not just calories, now it's time to hit the other half of the equation-exercise. Food has approximately 70% of the power to help you lose weight and maintain it. The other 30% is moving! I'm sure just hearing the word "exercise" is bound to make some people uncomfortable. Everyone who's ever tried to look for ways to lose extra pounds, whether it be from a web search or by asking their doctor, has virtually been told the same thing, that dieting and exercise are your two best shots! It's not just an annoying cliche; it actually holds a lot of truth behind it that no one can really deny. If you want to lose weight or keep it off, then you need to make exercise a regular part of your life. When you try to lose weight, the more you exercise, the more calories your body "burns off" or uses for energy.

When you cut back on the number of calories you eat and increase the number of calories you burn through exercise, this is called a "calorie deficit." A lot of evidence suggests that regular physical exercise is one of the best methods for maintaining low body weight, if not the best. Being in a calorie deficit while eating the proper percentages and quantities of Macros along with moderate exercise is the key to lifelong weight loss and maintenance. Aerobic exercise, also known as cardio, is a favorite among those looking to trim down. Many people like activities like walking, jogging, cycling, and swimming, for example, because they get the job done. But compared to lifting weights, aerobic exercises don't do much for your muscle growth. It burns calories quite well, though. (Donnelly et al., 2013) performed a 10-month study that looked at how exercising without dieting affected 141 adults who were obese or overweight. The test subjects were split into three groups, and they were not told to eat less. 4.3% of the participants burned 400 calories in each cardio session (5 times per week), and 5.7% of the participants burned 600 calories in each session (5 times per week) reducing body weight, respectively.

The exercise-free control group really put on 0.5% of their body weight. Several studies have also shown that cardio is a good way to lose body fat, especially the dangerous belly fat that is linked to a higher risk of type 2 diabetes and heart disease. So, if you keep your macros in the appropriate ratio and quantity and add exercise to your life, it will really help you lose weight faster. It will improve your metabolic health as well. The best combination I have found to actually lose weight after 40 is to food cycle. Do a period of time where you are at a lower macro quantity and not doing much exercise. A 20-minute walk per day is perfect. Then go through a period of time where you are both the food and the exercise. Build those muscles! Food Cycling is a great way to beat plateaus.

What Exercise Routine Is Best for You

The Physical Activity Guidelines for Americans say that people should do at least 150 minutes per week of moderate aerobic activity, 75 minutes per week of vigorous aerobic activity, or an equal mix of the two. So, the goal is to be active for 30 minutes at a moderate level five days a week. But I don't advise setting that objective right away for the majority of people, especially those who are new to exercising. Instead, gradually increase your activity level to create a habit that you can maintain. Creating and maintaining an exercise program requires serious mental work. If you set too high a goal for how long you want to work out, it might be hard to stay motivated. Start by working out for shorter amounts of time, like 5 to 10 minutes, so that your body can get used to the idea of regular exercise. Also, even a short session of exercise can improve your sense of self-worth, lift your spirits, and give you a sense of accomplishment. So, my standard advice is to take baby steps.

The biggest problem is getting into the habit of working out regularly, and five minutes a day can help you do that. You'll be surprised at how much better you feel after you've gotten into this routine. Consistently following a program is key to making it successful and yielding benefits. Always remember that, especially on those days when you really don't want to work out, and trust me, there will be those days, but you can do it! It's a shame that so many people who are new to working out get discouraged because they think they need to start off strong. No, it is entirely OK to begin at your own speed and have shorter workout durations. If you're just getting into the habit of jogging, for instance, don't force yourself to jog for an hour on the first day! All this will do is make you too exhausted to go running the following day since your body, which isn't acclimated to this new way of life, will be in shock and need time to adjust. Keep in mind that gradual and long-lasting growth is best. But if you can make a commitment, I suggest starting with 20 minutes of exercise every day.

A stroll, a run, yoga, stretching, Pilates, core work, or HIIT workouts are all excellent forms of exercise to start with. If you begin with 20 minutes, you will have sufficient time to warm up, reach your peak performance, and then transition into the cool-down phase. At some point, spending up to 30 minutes a day at least on working out is preferable, but my adage is that progress comes slowly but surely. Choose an activity goal that you can handle and stick with it. Once you've been able to commit to 20 minutes of activity every day for a few weeks, I suggest you fine-tune your workout plan by focusing on your goals. Most of the time, my clients are under a lot of stress and have excess belly fat. As a result, I advise picking an activity that reduces tension. Going on a stroll, working out with HIIT, or having fun by dancing while you exercise are all great options.

To Muscle up or Not to Muscle Up?

In a well-balanced recomposition of the body, losing weight and gaining muscle go hand in hand. When you lose weight and fat, especially in your stomach, your metabolism speeds up. This gives you the energy to train harder and build nice, lean muscles. Muscle, being the highly metabolically active tissue that it is, also helps with fat reduction. This is because our basal metabolic rate (BMR), or the number of calories your body burns at rest, increases as we gain muscle. So simply, the more muscle you have, the more fat you stand to lose. As I mentioned above, food cycling helps if you are both looking to lose weight and build muscle.

If you lose weight (also known as fat), you'll not only start to notice results sooner, but you'll also benefit from things like better sleep and a better mood. Although if you choose to prioritize muscle growth first, don't be surprised if you gain some weight in the early stages. In fact, you can count on this happening, but it shouldn't be a cause for concern. It's just that your muscle fibers are under stress from a new training routine. This results in some inflammation and tiny micro rips, commonly known as "microtrauma." This initial weight gain is what discourages a lot of women and may even lead some to give up on their good diet and exercise routines entirely. When you reduce your body fat percentage, you make your body's hormones more stable, which paves the way for improved insulin sensitivity and enhanced muscle-building potential (the way your body responds to and processes blood sugar).

When your primary goal is to build muscle mass, this will speed up your metabolism and make it easier to lose weight. Both are great goals. Strength training and eating more protein may help you keep as much muscle as possible while you lose fat and change the shape of your body by going after fat stores first. For long-term weight loss and fitness success, it's important to focus on both lowering body fat and building lean muscle mass. If you have a well-rounded plan for your workouts and food, you can reach both of your goals at the same time. But ultimately, your body fat percentage will determine this. So, if you're overweight or obese, which is defined as a body fat percentage of over 25% for men and over 32% for women, you should aim for weight loss first. And besides, it's way more difficult to try to grow muscle while also trying to cut body fat if you already have a lot of it. Your body will be more receptive to gaining muscle initially if you have a lower body fat percentage because you don't need to remove as much fat. You already know that losing weight has many advantages, including better sleep, lower blood pressure, lower risk of heart disease and diabetes, reduced blood sugar and cholesterol levels, and so forth. However, losing weight can also give you more energy and make you feel better about yourself overall. There will be less wear and tear on your ligaments and cartilage if you maintain a healthy body weight, which will make it easier to train hard and gain muscle.

The process of gaining muscle is often slower than the process of losing fat, which means that you will notice the effects of fat reduction much more quickly. If you focus on reducing your body fat first, you will be able to see your underlying muscle structure more clearly, which will make it easier for you to sculpt and define your physique. While it's true that building muscle may help you burn more calories because of the metabolic boost that comes with it, doing so takes time and a lot of work. Putting on muscle already takes women longer than males, so I would recommend shedding the pounds first before beginning to sculpt your beautiful physique. Gaining muscle mass increases your resting metabolic rate, which may be a significant help in the fight against obesity since it accounts for anywhere from 60-75% of our daily caloric expenditure. Putting forth the effort to eat a high-protein diet and work out in order to gain muscle mass is a double win for your waistline.

For instance, a study by (Longland et al., 2016) looked at individuals who consistently worked out hard and were in a caloric deficit. The study eventually concluded that those who consumed more protein lost 27% more fat and gained eight times as much lean muscle mass. Building muscle has many advantages beyond just boosting metabolism, though, including bettering your cardiovascular and joint health, lowering your risk of diabetes and certain cancers, enhancing your mental well-being, and enhancing bone health and strength, which reduces your risk of osteoporosis and falls. Whether you prioritize fat loss or muscle building depends on your unique health status and desired outcomes from your exercise program. To guarantee you're losing mostly fat and not hard-earned muscle, though, make sure your diet contains at least 0.7 grams of protein per pound of body weight (or 1.6 grams per kilogram). It's probably also a good idea to get someone like your accountability buddy to, well, keep you accountable. For best results, include enjoyable activities in your life. Ideally, this would include a mix of aerobic exercises, such as a HIIT workout, an interval workout, a long walk, or a run, as well as 2-3 days of strength training per week to maintain muscle mass. Strength training with heavier weights and fewer repetitions strengthens muscles, while aerobic endurance workouts like jogging, cycling, or brisk walking uphill improve stamina and allow you to train more often without tiring out. To promote muscle building, be sure to eat enough high-quality proteins throughout the day, with at least 20 grams of protein at each meal, such as fish, chicken, turkey, beans, lentils, and tofu. For the absolute best in a personalized macro and fitness program, you may reach me at www.lifelongmetaboliccenter.com.

Fact 6:

Habits to Hijack

There is no denying that humans are creatures of habit. We love following the same routine over and over again. For instance, most of us buy the same food every day from our "usual" supermarket and probably even cook the same meals, but if you want to become healthy and drop those pounds, you'll have to switch things up, abandon some of your unhealthy old routines, and adopt some new ways of thinking. The only issue is that we have a really hard time breaking old habits once we get used to them. People usually don't want to make positive changes to their diets because they are used to the foods and drinks they already eat and drink and are afraid of what might happen if they make these changes. Old habits are difficult to break, even when you know they're bad for you.

A habit is a learned behavior that develops through time and is stronger than a newer habit you are attempting to adopt." Even the most disciplined eaters can revert to old habits when under duress. When someone feels helpless or vulnerable, their instincts often take over, even if they want to do the right thing. Things may be going well until you reach a hard patch and are overcome by boredom, loneliness, sadness, or tension, which will have you reaching for those honey buns. Being self-aware is the first step to changing unhealthy eating and exercise habits.

The second step is to figure out why these habits started in the first place. The third step is to make a plan for making the necessary changes over time. By breaking the process into smaller pieces, you can make it easier to change your behavior in a way that will last. If you can make little changes over time, you'll soon be on the path to a healthier diet and a trimmer body. Changing to a healthy diet might be scary at first. However, success is more likely after you experience the positive effects of eating healthily and realize how delicious and nutritious food can be. If you stick with it, your taste for unhealthy foods will shift and eventually disappear.

Some habits I have taught my patients to ditch are stress eating through habit replacement, caving to cravings, and allowing yourself to keep your excuses. We covered habit replacement already. That's a MAJOR one. Cravings can be real or fake. Real cravings are when your body is sending you signals there is a need. One very common one is water. Another is fat. Fat makes you feel full, so if you have tried water, have a little healthy fat and see if it kicks that craving. Fake cravings may just be boredom or thinking about food. Change your mind and stomp those fake cravings. By disallowing your excuses, you can totally change your habits. Become a solution-finder rather than an excuse-maker. Every problem has a solution. Set your mind right and your body is soon to follow. If you find yourself unable to do this alone, there are amazing mental health professionals out there who are trained at retraining the brain. Reach out!

How To Change Your Habits

As the rock of life rolls along, we have gathered the "moss" of some bad habits. It's not too late to dump those and adopt new good habits. It takes three stages.

- Reminder (the trigger that triggers the action) This might be a deliberate action, like flushing the toilet, or a mood, like anxiety.

- Routine (the behavior itself that is related to the trigger; the action you execute): For example, flushing the toilet prompts you to wash your hands, while being anxious prompts you to bite your fingernails. Routine behavior may develop through repeated actions.

- Reward is the advantage gained from carrying out the activity (the benefit gained from carrying out the behavior). When there is a reward for an action, it becomes ingrained.

The "3 R's of Habit Change" concept has been repeatedly demonstrated by behavioral psychology experts. BJ Fogg, a Stanford professor, was the first to introduce me to the concept of habit formation. I learned about it in the latest edition of *The Power of Habit by Charles Duhigg*. The three phases of the "Habit Loop" are referred to as cue (reward), routine, and reward in Duhigg's book *How Habits Work* (Charles Duhigg, 2017). He says that almost any behavior can be changed with his techniques, though it might take some time and work. The structure is as follows: 1) figure out the routine (what needs to change), 2) try out different rewards, 3) find the cue, and 4) come up with a plan.

First, You Need to Pinpoint the Routine

In order to break a bad habit, you must first identify the feedback loop that keeps you engaging in it and then actively seek alternatives. Consider the following scenario: Say you've just clocked off from work, and you and your colleagues decide to go to a cafe to hang out and relax from the work day. This isn't anything new for you guys; in fact, you guys come to this particular cafe almost every day after work to enjoy some food, chat and laugh. All seems well and good until you realize that every time you're at this cafe, you have the nasty habit of purchasing a slice of their specially-made cheesecake (sometimes even more). Now, suppose you've put on some weight as a result of this routine. In fact, imagine this habit has led to an exact 11-pound weight increase. You have made several attempts to break this habit, even going so far as to write the words "no more cheesecake" on a post-it note that you pasted on your desk in an attempt to motivate yourself to quit. You see that letter every day before you leave the office, yet you still manage to accept your coworker's invitation, drive to the cafe, purchase that cheesecake, and indulge in it all the while conversing with coworkers at the seating section.

At first you feel great, you and your colleagues are sharing stories, enjoying good food, and just having a relaxing time overall after the work day. But after an hour when you all decide to go home, you start to feel guilty, and that good feeling turns into a regretful one. You feel great for a little while because of the dopamine receptors in your brain, but that all comes crashing down soon, and you end up feeling guilty. You make a commitment to yourself that you will have the willpower to resist tomorrow. It will be different tomorrow, but it never is, and the habit returns the next day. In order to begin correcting this habit, how do you identify it first? by identifying the habit loop of course. The first order of business is to recognize the pattern. The most obvious part of this cheesecake situation is the routine since it is the behavior you want to change.

Every day around five o'clock, you get up from your desk, make plans with your coworkers to meet up at the local cafe, where you enjoy a slice of cake while also having long and fun conversations with your work friends, and then repeat the next day. Thus, this is what you include in the loop. Following that, ask yourself several questions that may not be immediately apparent: What signals the start of this routine? Is it a drop in blood sugar? Boredom? Hunger? The cake itself? a shift in scenery? Stress from work? Stress at home? getting to know your coworkers? Or maybe that sugar rush that gives you a surge of energy? what is the prize? To find the answer, some trial and error will be required.

Experiment With Rewards in Step Two

The effectiveness of rewards lies in their ability to quell desires. However, we often aren't aware of the desires that motivate our actions. Most desires seem obvious when we look back on them, but it is very hard to tell when they are in charge of us. It helps to try out different rewards to figure out which cravings are behind certain behaviors. It's possible that this will take several days, up to a week, or even longer. During that time, you shouldn't put any pressure on yourself to make a significant adjustment; instead, you should see yourself as a researcher who is in the process of gathering information. When you sense the need to go to the cafe and purchase a cheesecake or any other dessert on the first day of your trial, change your routine so that it produces a new reward. For example, when you're at the cafe, instead of buying cheesecake, you could buy a coffee or a piece of fruit, eat it, then converse with friends before going home. Remember not to buy anything else but these two items. The next day, avoid going to the cafe altogether and instead go for an after-work jog or run with music. The next day, get your usual cheesecake. Then, as the next day rolls around, try something new, like a salad. Then the next day, instead of going to the cafe, you could invite a couple of your work friends somewhere else where there is no food that can tempt you. You get the gist.

It doesn't matter what you decide to do in place of purchasing that cake. Testing several theories can help you identify which desire is responsible for your pattern. Do you yearn for the desert itself? Are you just exhausted from work and need to unwind a little bit before going home? If so, go for a walk rather than giving in to the need to eat. Is the cake only a pretext for you to visit the cafe and mingle with your work friends? Did the workday tire you out and now you're in need of some energy in the form of sugar? (If yes, coffee or tea should be a better option.) Or are you really just hungry (in which case a salad or banana might also satisfy your hunger)? You may employ a tried-and-true method to search for trends as you try four or five different rewards: When you return home after each practice, write down on a piece of paper the first three ideas that spring to mind. They might be feelings, unrelated ideas, observations about how you're feeling, or even simply the first three words that come to mind. Next, set a 15-minute alarm on your computer or watch. When it sounds, ask yourself if you still want that piece of cake. Even if the three items are just words, it's still vital to record them for two reasons. It first compels you to briefly become aware of your thoughts and feelings.

Writing three words forces you to pay attention for a moment, just like how Mandy, the nail-biter in fact 3, carried around a note card with hash marks on it to make her aware of her repeated cravings. Additionally, studies demonstrate that jotting down a few words makes it easier to remember what you were thinking at the time in the future. It's particularly intriguing that taking notes seems to make crucial information easier for us to recall, and that the better our notes are, the more likely we are to do so. When you reread your notes at the conclusion of the experiment, your scrawled words will automatically produce a wave of remembering, and it will be much simpler to recall what you were thinking and experiencing at that precise time. And if you're wondering about the 15-minute alarm, it's because the goal of these tests is to identify the reward that you really want. If you still want the cake after chatting with coworkers, then your behavior probably isn't motivated by a need for human interaction. And if you still have the urge to go walk around while listening to music after eating your cheesecake, then your behavior isn't likely to be motivated by a sugar craving. But do notice if you really want to go get another slice of cake after those 15 minutes, because that's a sign of a sugar craving. But if you're happy with the end of your day after spending time with friends, even if you didn't have your piece of cake that night, that means you've found that "social engagement" is what your habit was looking for as a reward. Perhaps it was boredom and a need for a change of scenery that caused you to want human interaction, and that kind of socializing obviously centers around eating and chatting. So it's really easy to get sidetracked when in a conversation like this. But the good news is, you've identified the reward! To change a habit, you need to figure out what you really want, which you can do by practicing with different rewards. Knowing the pattern and the reward isn't enough to break the cycle; you also need to find out the cue, or "what is triggering you?"

Isolate the Cue in Step Three

A University of Western Ontario psychologist sought to solve a topic that has puzzled social scientists for years: why do some eyewitnesses of crimes misremember what they see? It goes without saying that eyewitness accounts are crucial. Despite this, research shows that eyewitnesses' memories are typically inaccurate. They claim that the killer had black hair and green eyes while, for example, he really had blonde hair and blue eyes. Others, however, have a near-perfect recollection of atrocities they saw as an eyewitness.

Researchers proposed two theories as to why some remember and others don't: either some individuals just have superior recollections, or crimes that take place in well-known settings are simpler to remember. However, such hypotheses were disproven because those with good and bad memory, or who were more or less acquainted with the scene of a crime, were equally likely to recall anything incorrectly. A distinct strategy was used by the

University of Western Ontario psychologist (Will, 2022). By concentrating on what interrogators and witnesses had said rather than how they were saying it, she questioned if academics were doing it wrong. She had a sneaking suspicion that there were subliminal indications dictating how the questions were asked. She searched through recordings and videotapes of witness interviews for these indicators, but she was unable to find any. She was unable to identify any trends since each interview was so chaotic due to the variety of facial expressions, questions asked, and emotions shown. So she had an idea: She produced a list of a few aspects she would pay attention to, including the tone of the questioner, the witness's facial expressions, and the distance between the witness and the questioner. She then deleted any material that would have drawn her attention away from those components. She reduced the television's volume so that she could only make out the tone of the questioner's voice rather than any spoken words. She covered the questioner's face with tape so that she could only see the witnesses' facial reactions. She measured their separation from one another by holding a tape measure up to the screen. And as soon as she began examining these particular components, patterns were obvious. She observed that officers often questioned witnesses who misremembered details in a kind, pleasant manner. The likelihood of misremembering increased when witnesses smiled more or sat closer to the person asking the questions. That is to say, eyewitnesses were more prone to distort the events that transpired when social indicators say "we are friends" (e.g., a soft tone, a kind expression). Maybe it was because such social signals made you want to satisfy the interrogator more than usual. However, what makes this experiment so significant is that hundreds of other researchers had already seen identical videos.

Although many intelligent individuals had seen the same correlations, no one had previously identified them. The reason was, each cassette had too much data to pick up on a slight hint. Except as soon as the psychologist made the decision to ignore all but three types of behavior and discard irrelevant data, the patterns were obvious. In many ways, our lives are identical. There is too much information coming at us as our behaviors develop, which is why it is so difficult to pinpoint the indicators that set off our habits. Is it hunger that drives you to have breakfast every morning at the same time? Or is it because it's 7:30? Or maybe it's because your kids are now eating? Or maybe you find that after you've gotten dressed, you have a greater tendency to eat breakfast. What motivates you to travel the same route to school every day even when you could go a different way? Is it the quickest path since there are the fewest roadblocks? or maybe it's all of the aforementioned? You're driving your child to school, but for some reason, you find yourself on the way to the office instead of the school's location. What was the trigger that made the habit of "driving to work" take hold instead of the habit of "driving to school"?

We may use the same method as the psychologist to pick out a signal from the background chatter by preparing ourselves to look for patterns in certain types of behavior. Fortunately, science may be of some assistance here. A majority of habitual cues, according to experiments, fall into one of five categories: location, time, other people, emotional state, and the action that comes right after it.

In order to identify the trigger for the habit of "going to the café and purchasing a cheesecake," you should note the following five factors as soon as the temptation strikes:

Where are you right now? (At the dining room table.) What is the time? (5:23 pm.) How do you feel at the moment? (happy that game night is taking place at the café.) Who else is in the area? (Katy, Ryan, Susie, and Michael.) What behavior came before the urge? (I wanted a cheesecake after seeing Susie enjoy one.)

Following day:

Where are you right now? (returning from my vehicle on foot.) What is the time? (5:18 pm.) How do you feel at the moment? (cheerful.) Who else is with you? (Michelle from accounting.) What behavior came before the urge? (Discuss office drama.)

Three days later:

Where are you right now? (Pier for businesses.) When is the time? (5:07 pm.) How are you feeling right now? (Excited to go unwind at the cafe despite being tired.) Who else is with you? (A few of my department's coworkers.) What behavior came before the urge? (The rest of the group is enthused.)

By day three, it ought to be obvious which cue sets off your habits. It was obvious which cue was setting off her cheesecake habit in the previous cheesecake example. She wanted social interaction and the rest of the day off from work as her reward. According to the day's example above, the habit trigger occurred between 5:00 and 6:00

Step 4: Create a plan.

You can start to change the behavior after you've recognized your habit loop, which includes the reward motivating your activity, the signal causing it, and the pattern itself. By anticipating the cue and adopting an action that will result in the desired reward, you may switch to a better pattern. You should make a plan. We discovered that habits are decisions that we make consciously at one time but then automatically repeat, usually on a daily basis. So basically, a habit is an instinctive pattern that our brain follows, such as when we perceive a cue, we will do a routine in order to get a reward. We need to start making decisions once again in order to re-engineer that formula. And several studies have shown that having a strategy is the simplest approach to do this. In psychology, these tactics are known as "implementation intentions." Consider the habit of eating cheesecake in the early evening. We were able to determine that the cue in that instance was about 5:30 in the afternoon by using this framework. The routine was to stroll down to the parking lot with the employees, drive to the café, get a cheesecake, take a seat, and talk with a friend for at least an hour. Through trial and error, we discovered (as she did) that what she truly craved was the chance to spend time with her friends and connect without having to worry about anything else for at least a little while, and that cheesecake was just an excuse.

I suppose you might argue that the benefit was a brief escape. Therefore, you need to record a strategy in your diary along these lines: If my friends suggest going to the café at around 5:00 p.m., I'll decline the offer and instead ask them if they want to go on a leisurely trek with me. Set an alarm for a few minutes before 5:00 to ensure that you remember to do this. This will allow you to leave and avoid walking to the parking lot with them if accepting their offer proves to be too alluring. If you have the choice, you might also park your vehicle on the other side of the parking lot to avoid encountering them before leaving to go home. Even if this may not work right away, continue with your strategy. There may be times (particularly early on) when your discipline still needs work, and you could stray from the path, but those are the times when you must keep your eyes on your goal and persevere! You'll discover that the end of the tunnel is not completely dark and that cheesecake has nothing on you. It goes without saying, however, that certain habits might be harder to break than others. But we can start with this foundation. Change might take a very long time. Repeated failures and experimentation are sometimes necessary. But you can control a habit once you know how it works—after you identify the signal, the pattern, and the reward.

Emotional Eaters

People who eat due to emotional ups or downs are what we call "emotional eaters." Is emotional eating something you struggle with? Do you ever find yourself reaching for, or desiring, a specific meal when you're upset, unhappy, bored, or lonely? As an example, after a long day of stress, an emotional eater may have a strong need for chocolate. And to be completely honest, I think it's safe to say that all of us are sometimes guilty of "eating our emotions." When feelings become overwhelming, it's not uncommon for people to seek solace in food. It's only human to look for stress relief methods after all. And since we depend on food for survival, eating is naturally gratifying. The problem is that relying on food as a form of stress relief or emotional support isn't exactly beneficial to one's physical or mental well-being. Naturally, your physical state will be impacted by your emotional eating habits. In addition to the obvious effects of gaining weight, overeating can also sap your vitality, trigger headaches, and otherwise make you feel awful. The other problem is that eating isn't effective as a means of dealing with negative feelings. While there is no shortage of advice on how to deal with emotional eating, it's important to note that severe dietary regimens don't suit everyone. Many of us continue to struggle with emotional eating even after we have learned and committed certain dietary rules to memory, such as restricting ourselves to one meal a day or not eating after 6 p.m. For sure, such was the situation with my pal Jessica. She is one of the funniest and most hardworking people I know. After all, being one of the best attorneys in her legal firm requires some effort.

This firm handles a lot of important cases for some of the most powerful people in the country, so Jessica is under a lot of pressure at work. It's not unusual for her to spend many nights working and fretting about work, and regrettably, the way she copes with this stress is to eat all of the pastries in the fridge. She confided in me that the only things that make her feel better whenever she is feeling stressed at work are sweets of any kind (ice cream, cupcakes, cinnamon buns, etc.). Of course, every time she finished a bar of chocolate, for instance, she would quickly feel the need for another item, and this would simply keep happening. "I'm not sure what's wrong with me. I know I should stop, but at those times, it's as if sweets are the only thing that can distract me from overthinking. "I feel like a failure," she said. I told her not to be so harsh on herself and explained that when you need food and then satisfy that craving, you receive an internal injection of Dopamine—a feel-good hormone. And that she ate a cookie every time she felt that unpleasant feeling—stress. Your brain's reward system is active, and you are content. However, this only lasts for a short time, and when you come down from that transient high and realize you're still agitated, you'll automatically grab for another cookie, and so the cycle repeats. Even if the goal of food rules is to promote self-control, it's not unexpected that they don't always end up being effective in the case of emotional eating. If you're an emotional eater like Jessica, you may think you have no control over what and how much you eat. In most cases, a person's emotional eating has nothing to do with a lack of willpower. In actuality, you most likely have lots of it! When it comes to eating out of emotional distress, it's rarely the act of eating itself that's the issue. Don't forget that humans are natural eaters! It's human nature to want something comforting to eat! Actually, the problem isn't with your eating habits per se, but with the unpleasant emotion that drives you to use food as a consolation. You're less likely to be able to stop emotional eating until you deal with the feeling that's driving you to eat in a way that is constructive and really helps you deal with the feeling.

To Help You Kick Emotional Eating:

1. Identify the Conduct

   Recognizing that you are engaging in emotional eating is the first step in overcoming this problem.

Learn to identify and accept emotional overeating for what it is so you may stop using food as a coping mechanism for emotions and start eating to satiate genuine hunger. What circumstances, locations, or emotions cause you to turn to food for comfort? Although it may sometimes be brought on by nice sensations, like rewarding oneself for reaching a goal or enjoying a special occasion, emotional eating is often associated with negative feelings. By realizing that the only reason you're eating right now is because you're feeling bad, you've already taken the first step toward getting rid of it. If you take the time to put your feelings into words on paper, you will have taken an even more significant step forward. This procedure may seem simple, even elementary. But in order to succeed in the long run, you must accept your conduct without criticizing yourself. The time has come to work very hard now. Here, judgment is not helpful to us. This just serves to exacerbate the problem. When you judge yourself harshly, you also experience intense feelings of shame and guilt, which only serve to increase your emotional burden and make it more difficult to work through your feelings. When you realize and accept that you are emotionally eating, remind yourself that you are a person who is feeling normal human emotions.

2. Find a way to deal with your emotional issue emotionally

When you want to stop stress eating or emotional eating, it helps to let yourself experience the emotion and then figure out a healthy way to deal with it. Like the example, we used above with the 3 R's. Now that you know what makes you turn to food when you're feeling down, you can go on to Step 2 and find a healthier way to deal with your emotions. Finding a more effective technique to deal with your feelings is the aim. Which begs the question: What is the best way to deal with your feelings? Well, this is a question that can only be answered on a case-by-case basis; here are some general suggestions for dealing with a range of typical emotions.

- Boredom: Try doing something different, like wrapping up an unfinished task, cleaning your house, or even just watching a movie or reading a book.

- Stress: breathing exercises, meditation, taking a quiet stroll, listening to calming music, and drinking water are all effective relaxation techniques.

- Anxiety: It might help to talk to a trusted friend, take a relaxing bath, play with your pet(s), or even see a professional. Even though it's true that some foods can help lower anxiety, it's best for people who have a problem with overeating to incorporate them into their diet rather than eat them on the spur of the moment because binge eating can actually make anxiety much worse from the food itself.

- Loneliness: Connect with friends or family by text, phone, or video chat.

- Sadness: try making a list of everything you're thankful for or watch a funny movie.

Trying to control your munching in the here and now is vital, but figuring out what's causing your stress in the first place is more crucial in the long run. Healthy routines like exercise, rest, and a balanced diet all serve as effective stress relievers.

3. Distinguish Between Emotional and Hunger Cues

   It's not always easy to tell the difference between eating because you're hungry and emotional eating. By eating consciously and paying attention to hunger cues, you may learn to distinguish between the two and control your eating. But, to put it simply, physical hunger builds up slowly and correlates with the time since your last meal. while factors like stress, anxiety, or weariness cause emotional hunger. Emotional hunger is often your body's way of letting you know that you need solace or something calming. Assessing your level of hunger on a scale of one to 10 is a good practice exercise. You may rank your level of hunger as anything between one and four if you're not really hungry, or just slightly so. Before eating, wait until you are actually hungry at five (but don't let yourself get extremely hungry to the point of overeating).

4. Establish a Schedule

Consistently adhering to a schedule of regularly spaced meals and, for some individuals, regularly spaced snacks, may help curb binge eating. Contrarily, erratic eating patterns are often problematic since they lead to impulsive and excessive eating. Some individuals plan their day around three main meals and two smaller meals, or "mini meals," spaced evenly throughout the day. The feeling of true hunger often sets in approximately three hours after the last meal. A little snack may be adequate at that point, depending on your eating habits and the time of day; if not, it's time for your next meal.

5. Replace With Healthy Behaviors

If you're used to eating in response to emotional situations, make a list of new habits to replace eating as a response to stress. They should take about 2-5 minutes, about the same amount of time as eating a snack. Some examples may be: soaking your feet in warm baking soda water, cleaning out a cabinet or closet, painting your nails, reading five pages in a book, etc. Do these, and you get the same dopamine "high" and a healthier outcome. When you retrain the habit of "stress eating" now, it will make keeping weight off later much easier. Walking is another easy, quick, and healthy substitute for emotional eating. You can walk normally, quickly, on a treadmill, or with your dog. Practicing a craft like knitting or felting not only provides a welcome diversion, they also provide an outlet for one's imagination and a means of making useful objects.

6. Examine Your Eating Habits

What you eat may not always matter as much as how you eat. More factors than just the particular items you choose to consume might contribute to emotional overeating, including overall food intake, attitude toward food, meal and snack balance, and individual eating patterns. Take stock of your eating habits, educate yourself on the differences between regular eating and emotional overeating, and come up with some new methods of self-help to deal with your mental and physical connections to food. It's important to practice saying "no" in order to succeed in forming healthier eating habits. This includes saying "no" to harmful meals as well as emotionally charged circumstances.

7. Change Your Eating Habits

Some individuals gain weight because they have unhealthy eating habits like skipping breakfast or eating late at night. But that doesn't mean you have to force yourself to have breakfast every morning, or that you can't eat anything at night if you really want to. But if your usual eating schedule isn't allowing you to slim down or keep your portions in check, you may want to try something different. Eating your major meal earlier in the day (for lunch) rather than later in the day (what may be considered conventional dinnertime) has been shown to aid with weight reduction and management in short-term trials. In other words, dine like a king (or queen) in the morning, and a princess (or beggar) in the afternoon.

8. Strike a Balance

In order to say that your life is well-balanced, you must be happy with all or almost all of its components. It implies that your physiological, psychological, and spiritual needs are being satisfied. A diet that is out of balance means that it either includes too few of the healthiest foods or too many of the unhealthiest ones. Emotional eating may also be a symptom of a deeper problem, such as a lack of self-care that manifests physically as illness, fatigue, or excess weight. Try to make changes in the parts of your life where you feel the most discontent in order to achieve a sense of equilibrium. Write these down. Score each section of your life and work on those with the lowest score first. This can help you keep from feeling overwhelmed and help to focus on one area at a time productively.

9. Collect Your Forces

Having a support system of loved ones and, if required, a therapist or coach may be just as crucial to your progress as your own drive and determination. Supporters can assist by encouraging you, suggesting better meal options, understanding the emotional roots of your overeating problems, and even assisting to defuse some of the emotional circumstances that cause your overeating. Create a support system of individuals who can listen, who can motivate, and inspire you, and who may even be willing to join you in your efforts to improve your health and wellness by cooking, walking, or working out. Social functions can make it difficult to stick to a diet, and if your life is rich in social outings, you will need a solution. Especially if someone in your life is a food pusher. Moms and grandmas are good at this. They often express love through food. In older generations, this may stem from a period in their own lives where food was scarce, so they don't want you to experience the same lack. Keep this in mind when responding. Enlist the help of someone else who will be with you at these functions. Kindly refuse and stick to your plan. It doesn't have to be dramatic or rude, but you will have to face it, so, this situation doesn't sabotage your progress.

10. Focus Inwards

You must always remind yourself that you are capable of completing any task at hand if you want to be successful. It's impossible to feel content and successful all the time; that's just not how life works. For instance, if you indulge in an emotional eating session, be kind to yourself and start again the next day. Make an effort to reflect on what went wrong and figure out what you can do to avoid this happening again. When you run into trouble, don't give up; instead, force yourself to keep looking for a way to solve the problem. Give yourself credit for the healthy lifestyle adjustments you've made, and keep your mind on the benefits of your new eating habits. While others may be of great assistance, it is up to you to identify your own abilities and utilize them to carry out the inner work and emotional work that you alone are capable of carrying out.

Fact 7:

Hunger Hacks

It's much easier said than done to eat healthily in order to lose weight. And if you've been trying to stick to a strict diet, you know how tempting it may be to revert to old eating habits. Some patients don't like keeping a food diary or skipping nightly ice cream while others don't see time in their schedule to exercise. One common issue is the feeling of hunger; not emotional eating, but truly feeling hunger. What, then, are some methods for regulating appetite and warding off unwelcome food cravings? It's crucial to keep in mind that using diet pills, herbal supplements, or crash diets to reduce weight might have detrimental long-term effects on your health. There are several natural methods you can use to help manage your hunger, but the first thing to do is determine if you are really, genuinely hungry in the first place.

How to Recognize When You're Really Hungry

Being "hungry" and "wanting something to eat" is not the same thing. You can tell the difference between real hunger and hunger caused by stress or emotions by a few clear signs. Start by answering the following questions: Is your tummy growling? Are you experiencing any "brain fog" or irritability? Have you seen a decrease in your energy levels? If you answered yes to any of these questions, you're probably experiencing real hunger. True hunger often manifests in these ways. In this state, your body is more likely to react positively to food, and you may experience an improvement in your mood after eating. Food, however, probably won't help you feel any less bored, angry, or sad if you're eating for reasons other than real hunger. And if it happens, you most likely won't experience that feeling for very long.

Best Techniques for Controlling Your Appetite

- *Get a lot of protein.* Consuming protein with each meal is a wonderful strategy to curb hunger pangs and eat less overall. In fact, among the three macronutrients (fats, carbohydrates, and protein), protein has been shown in several studies to have the greatest satiety-inducing effect. I always thought it was fat that was most satisfying and had read several studies stating that as well, so alas, we are back to getting a good balance of all three for the best results. These new studies say the hormone that causes hunger, ghrelin, is decreased by protein. Peptide YY, a hormone that makes you feel full, is also increased by it. These impacts on hunger may be quite potent. According to research that was conducted by (Weigle, 2022), increasing the amount of protein consumed from 15% to 30% of total calories caused overweight women to consume 441 fewer calories on a daily basis, even though they did not consciously limit anything. Foods that are high in protein are also low in calories per gram. Cutting down on carbs and fats may help you lose weight more quickly than cutting back on protein. It could be as easy as cutting down on the number of potatoes or grains you eat and adding a few more bites of fish or steak. You may also add foods like salmon, lean chicken, turkey, lentils, eggs, cottage cheese, Greek yogurt, and soybeans as high-protein meals.

- *Sip some coffee.* Both green tea and coffee have been shown to reduce hunger pangs and speed up the metabolic rate. But if you reach for these beverages, avoid those with excessive amounts of milk and/or sugar.

Some studies have shown that drinking coffee may help you eat less by reducing your hunger, delaying your stomach from emptying as quickly, and even influencing the hormones responsible for hunger. Plus, caffeine has been shown to promote fat-burning and support weight reduction. When caffeine is ingested, it increases the body's metabolism, thus temporarily reducing appetite. Thermogenesis, or the body's creation of heat and energy from the digestive processes, will be induced by caffeine. This means that for a short period of time, you will burn more calories because coffee encourages a stronger metabolic response from your body. In addition, compared to those who don't drink coffee, coffee drinkers may also be less prone to overeating during their next meal and throughout the day. It gives you something to sip on which fills your stomach and keeps your hands busy- also warm on cold winter days.

Eat plenty of high-fiber, water-rich meals to fill up. There are no calories in water or fiber. High-water-content meals with plenty of fiber are "bulky" and make you feel full because they take up more room in your stomach. Also, due to their high water and fiber content, the majority of vegetables—aside from those that are starchy like potatoes, corn, and peas—have relatively few calories per serving. You can also feel full at a relatively cheap calorie cost by eating watery fruits like melons and pineapple as well as rich fiber foods like berries.

Eat a lot of nuts. Protein, unsaturated fat, vitamin E, magnesium, and antioxidants are all abundant in nuts. If you're feeling hungry, grab a handful, and you'll soon forget you were hungry. Beware though of the serving size of nuts. They, along with nut butters are easy to overeat. By purchasing single-serving packets, you can eliminate overeating. Another tip is to get whatever serving size you intend to eat, close the container, and walk away before you start eating. Then you are less likely to go back to the room and reopen the container for more. Even if you do, you burned extra calories and got extra steps by having to go back to the kitchen.

- *Add spice to your food.* Spices that help boost your metabolism and curb your hunger include cayenne pepper, black pepper, turmeric, cinnamon, and curry. Cayenne pepper, for instance, has been shown to help the body burn more fat when eaten with high-carb meals.

- *Consume more omega-3 fatty acids.* The hormone leptin, which causes a sensation of fullness after eating, is increased by the omega-3 fatty acids contained in fish, making them especially effective at lowering appetite.

- *Do not chew gum regularly or for extended periods of time.* The act of mastication (chewing) tells your body that food is on the way, so it speeds digestion up and makes you hungrier sooner than you otherwise may have been. For breath freshening, sip mint herbal teas or try the breath strips or sprays.

- *Pay attention to your urges for snacks.* If you ignore your hunger, it's possible that you'll overeat when it's time for a meal, which will make your hunger worse. Choose healthy options like hummus, carrot sticks, fruit, etc. whenever you feel like nibbling so you can help keep yourself full without consuming a lot of calories. If you are watching your macros, plan snacks that fit what you need for the day ahead of time. Then you can hit what your body needs, curb hunger before it hits, and not really have to give any time or thought to food on a daily basis-just once a week or so for planning time.

- *Sip on liquids to help you feel fuller longer.* Having a beverage with your meal may help you feel fuller with less food. Unfortunately, some individuals eat when they really need to drink water because they misinterpret their body's signals. That's less likely to occur if you drink plenty of water all throughout the day and with each meal.

- *Exercise is a great way to curb your appetite.* Exercise helps reduce your appetite by suppressing hunger hormones. Of course, you can't keep going if you don't give your body the nourishment it requires. A person's efforts to lose weight may backfire if they severely restrict their caloric intake and become too exhausted to keep up with their regular exercise routine. Therefore, the whole operation fails. Some of my patients have complained to me that physical activity just makes them hungrier and causes them to overeat. However, this is usually the result of inadequate pre- and post-workout nutrition.

- *Small, regular meals might help you control your hunger.* Eating modest, frequent meals throughout the day helps maintain more steady blood sugar levels. This is crucial since spikes in appetite can be brought on by drops in blood sugar. Even if you're worried that a smaller meal won't be enough to satisfy your hunger, knowing that you'll be able to refuel in a few hours could be extremely helpful. Others find that intermittent fasting is actually best for their body and hunger. Stay with me here, but for some not starting to eat for the day cause their appetite to not kick in yet. They report (and studies show) that intermittent fasting causes your body to burn your own fat stores when done properly. When you switch over to fat-burning mode, there is plenty of energy and no hunger. Some do intermittent as in 18 hours with no food, then 6 hours of eating or something equivalent. Others do 24 hr fasts weekly or bi-weekly.

- *Use dark chocolate to satisfy your sweet cravings.* Dark chocolate should be chosen over milk chocolate if you have a serious sweet tooth. When the cocoa content is 75% or 80% or above, there is less sugar and more room for moderation. Read research, talk with your doctor, and decide if "grazing" or intermittent fasting may be a better solution for your body and your lifestyle. Before you write them off, give them each a good try. You may be surprised at which one works best for your body. My favorite, as I mentioned earlier, is food cycling-a combination of the two. It seems to be a real plateau buster for most.

A Useful Method to Try

Okay, so let's say that you've followed every piece of advice I offered in this book, and now you have regular meals and maybe even scheduled snacks, or you are absolutely rocking intermittent fasting. During the first week of your new lifestyle, you may experience some mild symptoms, like hunger. Don't worry; this is typical. Because your body is still adapting to this new "normal," the first week or two of a new diet is usually the most difficult. Just remember to stick to your plan, and you won't just lose weight but also find that you're not as hungry as you were before after a few weeks. This is because you will be conditioning your body to anticipate meals only at certain times of day and in smaller amounts. However, the first two weeks may make or break a diet, so here's what I advise doing if those pesky hunger cues appear:

1. Drink

   Drinking 16 ounces of water (two cups) causes your stomach to expand, which signals your brain that you are no longer hungry. It's also ideal to consume these two cups at least 30 minutes before you plan to eat. This is because when you think about eating, your mouth starts to salivate and your stomach starts making digestive fluid to get ready for the meal. If you drink water just before eating in such a condition, your saliva and digestive secretions will dissolve. And since we already know that drinking water makes you feel full, you'll naturally consume fewer calories overall. You'll soon feel hungry again once the water has been absorbed, which might lead to overeating. Since most individuals mistake hunger for thirst, this approach is also helpful in determining whether you are indeed hungry. After drinking 16 ounces of water and waiting 15 minutes, you should find that your hunger pains have gone away. If they haven't, you're probably really hungry, in which case I recommend the next step.

2. Do Deep Breathing Exercises and Wait for 15 Minutes

    To do breathing exercises, all you have to do is concentrate on your breathing while shutting off the world around you-easy, right? LOL. Deep breathing specifically is a kind of breathing exercise that entails taking a deep breath, holding it for a little while, and then slowly exhaling it. Every one of us has probably heard that regular breathing exercises help people relax, feel better, and concentrate more effectively. Because of this, it seems likely that doing breathing exercises regularly is good for mental health and, by extension, our quality of life. Fewer people, on the other hand, know how good it is for our physical health. When you train your breathing muscles on a daily basis, you not only improve your health but also reduce your appetite and increase your feelings of fullness. This helps you maintain a healthy weight by preventing you from eating too much. This impact of breathing exercises on appetite regulation was discovered in a study by (Voroshilov, 2017). The study specifically linked Qigong breathing exercises to improved appetite regulation. Qigong includes many ways to regulate appetite by bringing the body and mind into harmony. Standing is the best way to do the exercise, or modified standing with the body leaning forward and both upper limbs resting on a countertop. Ideally, standing upright with your feet shoulder-width apart and your hands either on your stomach or along the length of your body is the starting position. Draw your stomach in while taking a deep breath and straightening your shoulders. For three to four seconds, you should hold your breath while holding your stomach in and using your ab muscles to their fullest extent to retract your stomach muscles. As you exhale, your chest and abdominal muscles will relax, and your shoulders will return to their initial posture. At a minimum, you should do this exercise 10–15 times. If you are overweight and find it difficult to pull in your stomach while standing, you can perform this exercise while sitting and supporting yourself with both hands. While we're talking about the respiratory system, it's important to note that breathing with your diaphragm has been shown to speed up your metabolism. And because we all know that women in this stage of life have a slower metabolism, this may be the ideal solution for us gals over 40. This is brought on by the body's altered hormonal balance. That makes gaining weight much easier but losing weight much more difficult. This breathing method may help reduce stress eating, cortisol levels and aid in a quicker metabolism. Triple threat! In cases where the issue isn't how many calories you're consuming, calorie restriction won't always lead to weight reduction, but this breathing method may. This was demonstrated in a study by (Yong et al., 2018), in which half of the 38 participants engaged in diaphragmatic breathing. This is also called "belly breathing," and it means taking in enough air to stretch your diaphragm. The muscle that looks like a dome and is right above your stomach and below your lungs is called your diaphragm. The other half used feedback breathing devices to practice alternative breathing techniques. Researchers discovered a substantial difference in total oxygen intake and resting metabolic rate in the diaphragmatic breathing group. These benefits were not seen in the other group utilizing the breathing apparatus. The following is a guide for practicing diaphragmatic breathing:

- With your legs bent and a low pillow under your head, lie on your back on a yoga mat or in bed. If more support is required, put a cushion beneath your knees.

- Put one hand slightly below your ribcage on your abdomen, and the other on your upper chest.

- Inhale deeply through your nose and feel the air settle into your torso and belly. At first, keep your hand motionless on your chest while raising your belly hand.

- As you gently exhale through pursed lips, tighten your abdominal muscles and allow them to go inward toward your spine. Return the hand to its previous position on your belly.

Spend at least 10 minutes a day using this breathing method to get more energy, a faster metabolism, lower blood pressure, and an easier time losing weight. Though it may take some extra work to get the hang of using your diaphragm properly at first, you'll quickly see the benefits of putting in the time and effort. Once you know how to do it, try it while sitting in a chair with your knees bent and your shoulders, head, and neck in a comfortable, neutral position, or you can just sit on your floor mat with your legs crossed as part of your yoga or other workout routines. Wait another 15 minutes after you've finished your breathing exercise before moving on to the next phase if hunger is still on your mind.

3. Eat a High Fiber Food

Pair a high-fiber food like celery with Pink Himalayan salt, or almond butter. Consume citrus fruits like oranges and grapefruits since they are high in soluble fiber and low in calories. These types of foods are fantastic for satiating appetites since they make us feel full more quickly and keep our blood sugar levels constant. I only propose oranges or grapefruit since they have the greatest fiber content among the top 20 fruits and vegetables, but it doesn't have to be those two. Oats, which are low in calories and have a lot of both soluble and insoluble fibers, are another good choice. The soluble fiber beta-glucan in oats keeps you feeling full for longer. This is one reason why oats are so popular as a breakfast food. A green salad would be a great choice as well since it's also very rich in fiber and you can top it with celery sticks. Celery sticks have a crunch that is comparable to that of chips or crackers, which makes them an excellent snack in general. Celery is also rich in water content, low in calories, and high in fiber. Now Include some Pink Himalayan salt for flavor and to increase its appetite-suppressing effects. Historically, Himalayan salt has been used in both Ayurvedic and TCM treatments. It has become popular in many health communities because of the health benefits it is said to have during intermittent fasting, such as more energy and a smoother digestive system. By increasing blood flow to your stomach, pink salt reduces hunger sensations by decreasing the amount of blood that travels there. Alternatively, if you don't want to eat more salt, I suggest adding a tiny bit of almond butter. Almond butter has a decent quantity of fiber and healthy fats, which may help you feel fuller for longer. You won't feel the need for a snack in between meals since it helps control your appetite. This is useful if you're trying to control or lose weight and are spacing out your meals and keeping an eye on your food consumption.

The Recap

Yay, you've made it to this part of the book! I am a gal who does not like to waste time-mine or anyone else's, so I wanted this book to have a quick reference section with just the bullet points of the important stuff. You've read the studies and digested the details (pun intended), now here is the "meat and potatoes" of how-to. Okay so first thing is water, the following should help:

Put Some Flavor in It

If you don't like the way water tastes or if you find drinking water dull, this is a fantastic alternative. Mix some fruit into your water. Citrus fruits like oranges, lemons, and limes have already been tried and tested-delish! Some more tasty alternatives are cucumbers, watermelons, berries, and mint. These can also make the drink pretty, and thus more fun to drink!

Eat It

Melons, cucumbers, lettuce, and celery are just a few examples of the many fruits and vegetables that are mostly composed of water, which makes it simpler to consume more water without realizing it. There are also a variety of soups, popsicles (though be careful with the sugar content), and smoothies to choose from (again watch the sugar here.)

Incorporate It Into Your Daily Schedule

Every time you clean your teeth, before you eat a meal, or before you enter the kitchen, drink a glass of water. One might find this approach to be very helpful. Because of this, I've been drinking a lot more water, and it has improved so much more than just my weight. I can't remember the last time my skin looked this glowy!

Follow It

The best way to keep track of your water intake is with a smart water bottle that syncs with your phone. Alternatively, you could use a calendar or alarm to keep tabs on your consumption.

Vary Your Beverage Choices

If you can't give up sugary drinks totally, try diluting them with water. When you've had enough water for the day, drink some soda or juice instead as a rare treat.

Grab It and Go

When you're always on the go, it might be hard to remember to take in enough fluids, therefore if you want to stay hydrated throughout the day, fill up a water bottle before you leave the house and carry it with you everywhere you go.

The Best Way to Kickstart Your Food Journaling Journey

Be gentle with yourself as you adapt, and try to be as consistent as you can. It's likely to be effective if it seems tough yet doable. Don't worry yourself sick if you miss a day here and there. Simply pick it back up right away. Just remember that this is a temporary state and it too shall pass. Keeping a food diary for a year or just today might teach you a lot about your eating habits. While the tried-and-true method of using a pen and piece of paper is still viable, it may not be for you. Take some images, use an app, or try writing something down on your phone to find the best option for you. That being said here are some tips I find useful for those new to journaling:

1. Don't Leave Anything Out of Your Record, Even if It's "Only a Taste."

   Even if you record every single meal and snack you have, your food diary won't be accurate if you don't also record the little, unnoticed bites of food and drink you have. Here are some examples, Say You're making dinner for the entire family, and you keep tasting it as you go to make sure it's not too salty or too sweet. Or, every time you pass by the office cafeteria, you swipe for a sweet dessert, or when you'd normally drink black coffee, but you choose to add creamer and sugar today. Note these events as they happen to ensure that your efforts are in line with your objectives, such as weight reduction or muscle building. Writing it down on the notes app on your phone and transferring it later to your diary is also an excellent strategy. These types of minor tastes are rather simple to quantify. If you decide to add half-and-half to your coffee, for instance, you may base your entry on the fact that one tablespoon of half-and-half has 20 calories. Write down your estimate of how much more you poured. In the grand scheme of things, the extra 20 calories from coffee cream won't matter, but if you're always nibbling and not recording, your diary will become inaccurate, and you'll be left wondering why you haven't accomplished your objectives.

2. Recognize Serving Sizes

For the first several weeks of keeping a food diary, you should measure meals exactly if you are unfamiliar with serving sizes. If you've never kept a food diary before, it's a good idea to get a food scale so you don't accidentally under-or overestimate your portions. All you need is an affordable food scale that you can get from the grocery store or a simple scale from Target. Eventually, you'll be able to forgo measuring cups and spoons in favor of winging it. Example: A deck of cards is roughly the same size as three ounces of protein. A ping pong ball is roughly the size of a two-tablespoon dollop of nut butter. The size of a teaspoon is comparable to a dice.

3. Give Detailed, Honest Information

Don't try to sugarcoat (I'm so punny) or otherwise alter what you ate in order to avoid feeling guilty; instead, record it precisely as it happened. For instance, don't be cheeky and simply type "potato" if you had fried chips. You'll go nowhere in the long term because this is too vague and lacks specificity. The terms "potato" and "fried chips" have quite distinct macronutrient profiles, so using them interchangeably won't help you monitor your nutrition.

4. Record the three Ws, including who, where, and when.

When did you eat, where did you eat, and who was there with you when you did? Our food consumption and dietary preferences are profoundly affected by all of these factors. Personally, I know that when I eat while watching TV, I consume much more calories than when I eat while seated at the table. It's possible that this is the case because I feel more at ease on the sofa since it's a less formal atmosphere and I can just chill. But I also know that I tend to overeat when I am in the company of others, most likely because I am too preoccupied with conversing and enjoying the company of others to notice that I am eating.

5. Snap Pictures

With our busy lives, the human memory isn't always as impressive as it could be. We are scattered and fragmented on a daily basis. You can easily fool yourself into believing a falsehood since our mental file cabinets are very prone to errors and forgetfulness. For this reason, it's recommended that, in addition to recording your meals in a diary, you also take photographs of them. Pictures tell a thousand words, plus it's always interesting to go back and examine how one's eating habits have changed over time.

Here Are Some Pointers for Maintaining a Regular Exercise Schedule

- **Aim for Something**

  Prioritize setting short-term objectives before moving on to longer-term ones. Ensure that your objectives are doable and realistic. If your objectives are too lofty, it'll be easy to lose motivation and give up. In the event that you haven't worked out in a while, a reasonable short-term objective may be to stroll for 10 minutes, five days a week. Of course, exercise, no matter how brief, has advantages. Aiming to get in 30 minutes of walking five days a week is a reasonable intermediate step. To walk five kilometers (~3 miles) would be a worthy long-term objective.

- **Make It Enjoyable**

  If you want to stay motivated, it's important to choose an activity or sport that you like doing and then mix it up. Exercise should be fun, so if you're not having fun, you should switch things up. Try out for a local softball or volleyball team. Learn some ballroom dance moves. Try visiting a nearby gym or dojo (or krav maga studio). You can find recordings of many other sorts of workout courses, including yoga, HIIT, and kickboxing, online if you want to work out in the comfort of your own home. Alternatively, you may go for a jog or a stroll at a nearby park. Learn about any latent sports hobbies or skills you may possess. Exercise need not be monotonous, and if you like it, you are more likely to persist with a fitness program.

- **Document It**

  Put your objectives on paper. If you can clearly see yourself reaping the benefits of regular exercise and write down your goals, you may find it easier to stay motivated. Keeping an exercise journal could just be what you were missing. Maintain a journal detailing your workouts, how long they lasted, and how you felt afterward. Keeping a log of your efforts and accomplishments might encourage you to keep pushing forward toward your objectives.

- **Include Exercise in Your Everyday Regimen**

  Finding time to exercise might be challenging, but that's no reason to put it off. To be effective, physical exercise must be planned ahead of time, just like any other mandatory task. Regular exercise can be integrated into your day in little increments. For example, Rather than using the elevator, make it a thing to start using the steps instead. Or as you watch the children play sports, stroll up and down the sidelines. Get some fresh air and exercise during your company's break time by going for a stroll, etc. It's especially important for those who work from home to take frequent breaks to get up and move about. Alternatively, you can perform sit-ups, lunges, and squats. Go for a walk with your dog if you have one.

Spend your lunch break or evenings in front of the TV doing some strength training routines, such as pedaling a stationary bike or walking/jogging on a treadmill. While doing the necessary amount of exercise each week is important for good health, studies show that sitting for lengthy periods of time might have a detrimental impact on health. If your profession requires you to sit for long periods of time, try to include short periods of movement throughout your day. This might be as simple as getting up to grab a sip of water or as involved as standing up during phone calls or online conferences.

- **Treat Yourself**

Make sure you allow yourself some time after each workout to bask in the glow of satisfaction. Motivating yourself in this way might help you maintain your fitness routine over time. Other incentives may also be good. Reward yourself with a new pair of walking shoes or some new music to listen to as you walk after you meet a long-term fitness goal.

- **Be Adaptable**

    If you're sick, overworked, or just plain tired, you're allowed to skip a day or two from your usual regimen. Relax your standards if you feel like you need a break without criticizing yourself too harshly. The most crucial thing anyway is to quickly resume your original course of action as soon as you can. Get going after your energy has returned! Set your own objectives, have fun with it, and sometimes give yourself a pat on the back. Never underestimate the value of exercise. If you find your drive waning again, revisit these suggestions.

How to Get Motivated to Start Working When You're Having Mental Issues

For good reason, the adage "getting started is the hardest part" is often used. The motivation needed to start any endeavor might be far higher than the motivation needed to complete it after you've gained momentum and concentration, whether it's exercising, regularly writing, attempting to control your emotional eating, etc. Even the most basic actions, like remembering to drink water or maintaining your resolve and resisting the urge to go for that muffin, may seem plain hard if you are also feeling anxious or cognitively challenged that day. Fortunately, the advice I provided you in the chapters above on how to deal with stress or emotional upheaval should be able to help you out sufficiently. However, I just wanted to give a brief refresher and a few more tips on how to make your first week a little bit easier. So, If you're having difficulties getting things done, whether it's your to-do list or your day-to-day obligations, try one of these methods to rekindle your drive.

Make A Plan. Work The Plan

Having a pile of unorganized tasks to complete staring you in the face is a certain way to put you in a funk and make whatever issue you're already facing much more difficult to handle. In such a scenario, time management is crucial. You should sit down for a period of time each day, and document/organize before starting the everyday activities. (Or do this once per week for the whole week). Exercise in the morning, complete important tasks in the first three hours so that you can rest after your workday is through, take a stroll around your building at lunch to get some fresh air, and so on are some examples. Whatever way you choose to organize it, be sure to reserve certain times of the day for certain duties. Making a schedule for your day helps you feel a lot more in control of your responsibilities. You may use your phone's calendar with notifications to remind you when to switch tasks, or a specific app.

Take Everything Step-By-Step

To avoid feeling overwhelmed, break down each item on your list into smaller, ostensibly more manageable chores. You'll get a dopamine rush as you check each item off the list. I promise you'll feel great about yourself for getting things done like when you do all the exercises you set out to do in a single session or refrain from overeating. By breaking up longer tasks into shorter bursts, you can get a lot done. Although it won't last long, this impact will provide you with just enough motivation to get you through those times when you're not feeling driven. No matter how much you may believe you are capable of, it is easier to motivate yourself when you have little, short tasks to do.

Compile an Inspiring Playlist

Lots of individuals, including myself, have a go-to playlist for when we need to buckle down and get through a tough endeavor. Certain types of music have the ability to truly motivate you to take action. It might be easier to be in the correct frame of mind and even feel more at ease when you're feeling off, uninspired, or just plain worried if your work area has a regular background. If you have a favorite playlist, whether it's one you made yourself or one you found on Spotify or YouTube, it's best to stick to it. Put in some fresh tunes every so often to keep things interesting.

Don an Attractive Outfit

This may sound strange, vain, or superficial, but there is truth to it. Clothing and accessories may help you feel more confident and put together when you're feeling overwhelmed by life's stresses. Putting on an item of clothing that makes you feel really good about yourself may be a great confidence booster. Even if you don't feel like working out today, putting on some nice exercise attire will help spark some enthusiasm. Wake up, get up, dress up, show up.

Conclusion

So, to recap and leave you with knowledge, empowerment, and encouragement: As we get older, it gets harder to keep weight off for a variety of reasons, such as stress, hormones, a slower metabolism, and so on. Even so, that doesn't mean that nothing can be done about it. The goal of this book was to show you how to lose weight after age 40 in a healthy way. I intended to demonstrate weight loss and weight maintenance FACTS, which is why the chapters were labeled as they were. I wanted the book to leave you with a sense of optimism and hope, not simply instructions for doing the thing. Instead of becoming disheartened, I want you to rise to the challenge by using the simple strategies offered in this book. I want you to accept that this is NOT your new normal and do something about it. You may have thought that there's no hope for regaining the weight-loss success you had at age 25, but if you're willing to put in the effort and follow a good strategy, you won't have to worry about your weight again. Whether your goal is to increase your water intake, raise your level of self-awareness, increase your daily step count, or increase your vegetable consumption, the key is to simply get started and keep going. Humans are hardwired to respond more strongly to negative feelings like self-doubt and self-pity, but I can promise you that these are merely your cavewoman brain's attempt to keep you feeling "secure" and comfortable. When you hear it, tell it to get lost and remind yourself, "I can do anything I put my mind to!" because, well, you are amazing! Now that you're equipped with this knowledge and revved up, there's no better time to start. If you have enjoyed this book and learned some tips and tricks to make your life healthier, please leave me a review on Amazon.

References

Berg, J. (2021, August 31). Tamra Judge Is Done with the Keto Diet: *"I gained weight."* Bravo TV Official Site; Bravo. https://www.bravotv.com/the-real-housewives-of-orange-county/style-living/tamra-judge-stops-keto-diet-after-weight-gain

Boschmann, M., Steiniger, J., Hille, U., Tank, J., Adams, F., Sharma, A. M., Klaus, S., Luft, F. C., & Jordan, J. (2003, December 1). *Water-induced Thermogenesis.* The Journal of Clinical Endocrinology & Metabolism, 88(12), 6015–6019. https://doi.org/10.1210/jc.2003-030780

Brown, C. M., Dulloo, A. G., & Montani, J.-P. (2006, September 1). Water-Induced Thermogenesis Reconsidered: *The effects of Osmolality and water temperature on energy expenditure after drinking.* The Journal of Clinical Endocrinology & Metabolism, 91(9), 3598–3602. https://doi.org/10.1210/jc.2006-0407

Castro-Sepulveda, M., Ramirez-Campillo, R., Abad-Colil, F., Monje, C., Peñailillo, L., Cancino, J., & Zbinden-Foncea, H. (2018, September 26). *Basal mild dehydration increase salivary cortisol after a friendly match in young elite soccer players.* Frontiers in Physiology, 9. https://doi.org/10.3389/fphys.2018.01347

Corney, R. A., Sunderland, C., & James, L. J. (2015, April 18). *Immediate pre-meal water ingestion decreases voluntary food intake in lean young males.* European Journal of Nutrition, 55(2), 815–819. https://doi.org/10.1007/s00394-015-0903-4

Davy, B. M., Dennis, E. A., Dengo, A. L., Wilson, K. L., & Davy, K. P. (2008, July). *Water Consumption Reduces Energy Intake at a Breakfast Meal in Obese Older Adults.* Journal of the American Dietetic Association, 108(7), 1236–1239. https://doi.org/10.1016/j.jada.2008.04.013

Dehghan, M., Mente, A., Zhang, X., Swaminathan, S., Li, W., Mohan, V., Iqbal, R., Kumar, R., Wentzel-Viljoen, E., Rosengren, A., Amma, L. I., Avezum, A., Chifamba, J., Diaz, R., Khatib, R., Lear, S., Lopez-Jaramillo, P., Liu, X., Gupta, R., & Mohammadifard, N. (2017, November 04). Associations of fats and carbohydrate intake with cardiovascular disease and mortality in 18 countries from five continents (PURE): *a prospective cohort study.* The Lancet, 390(10107), 2050–2062. https://doi.org/10.1016/s0140-6736(17)32252-3

Donnelly, J. E., Honas, J. J., Smith, B. K., Mayo, M. S., Gibson, C. A., Sullivan, D. K., Lee, J., Herrmann, S. D., Lambourne, K., & Washburn, R. A. (2013, March 21). Aerobic exercise alone results in clinically significant weight loss for men and women: *Midwest exercise trial 2.* Obesity, 21(3), E219–E228. https://doi.org/10.1002/oby.20145

Garcia-Navarro, L. (2018, April 29). "Tully Gets It": *Charlize Theron Wants An Honest Conversation About Motherhood.* NPR.org. https://www.npr.org/2018/04/29/606062105/tu lly-gets-it-charlize-theron-wants-an-honest-conver sation-about-motherhood

Harland, J. I., & Garton, L. E. (2008a, June 11). *Whole-grain intake as a marker of healthy body weight and adiposity.* Public Health Nutrition, 11(6), 554–563. https://doi.org/10.1017/s1368980007001279

Harland, J. I., & Garton, L. E. (2008b, June 11). *Whole-grain intake as a marker of healthy body weight and adiposity.* Public Health Nutrition, 11(6), 554–563. https://doi.org/10.1017/s1368980007001279

Hollis, J. F., Gullion, C. M., Stevens, V. J., Brantley, P. J., Appel, L. J., Ard, J. D., Champagne, C. M., Dalcin, A., Erlinger, T. P., Funk, K., Laferriere, D., Lin, P.-H., Loria, C. M., Samuel-Hodge, C., Vollmer, W. M., & Svetkey, L. P. (2008a, August). *Weight Loss During the Intensive Intervention Phase of the Weight-Loss Maintenance Trial.* American Journal of Preventive Medicine, 35(2), 118–126. https://doi.org/10.1016/j.amepre.2008.04.013

Hollis, J. F., Gullion, C. M., Stevens, V. J., Brantley, P. J., Appel, L. J., Ard, J. D., Champagne, C. M., Dalcin, A., Erlinger, T. P., Funk, K., Laferriere, D., Lin, P.-H., Loria, C. M., Samuel-Hodge, C., Vollmer, W. M., & Svetkey, L. P. (2008b, August). *Weight Loss During the Intensive Intervention Phase of the*

Weight-Loss Maintenance Trial. American Journal of Preventive Medicine, 35(2), 118–126. https://doi.org/10.1016/j.amepre.2008.04.013

Hollis, J. F., Gullion, C. M., Stevens, V. J., Brantley, P. J., Appel, L. J., Ard, J. D., Champagne, C. M., Dalcin, A., Erlinger, T. P., Funk, K., Laferriere, D., Lin, P.-H., Loria, C. M., Samuel-Hodge, C., Vollmer, W. M., & Svetkey, L. P. (2008c, August). *Weight Loss During the Intensive Intervention Phase of the Weight-Loss Maintenance Trial.* American Journal of Preventive Medicine, 35(2), 118–126. https://doi.org/10.1016/j.amepre.2008.04.013

How Habits Work - Charles Duhigg. (2017, November 20). Charles Duhigg. https://charlesduhigg.com/how-habits-work/

Longland, T. M., Oikawa, S. Y., Mitchell, C. J., Devries, M. C., & Phillips, S. M. (2016, January 27). *Higher compared with lower dietary protein during an energy deficit combined with intense exercise promotes greater lean mass gain and fat mass loss: a randomized trial.* The American Journal of Clinical Nutrition, 103(3), 738–746. https://doi.org/10.3945/ajcn.115.119339

Madjd, A., Taylor, M. A., Delavari, A., Malekzadeh, R., Macdonald, I. A., & Farshchi, H. R. (2015, November 4). Effects on weight loss in adults of replacing diet beverages with water during a hypoenergetic diet: *a randomized, 24-wk clinical trial.* The American Journal of Clinical Nutrition, 102(6), 1305–1312. https://doi.org/10.3945/ajcn.115.109397

Morita, Yokoyama, Imai, Takeda, Ota, Kawai, Hisada, Emoto, Suzuki, & Okazaki. (2019a, April 17). *Aerobic Exercise Training with Brisk Walking Increases Intestinal Bacteroides in Healthy Elderly Women.* Nutrients, 11(4), 868. https://doi.org/10.3390/nu11040868

Morita, Yokoyama, Imai, Takeda, Ota, Kawai, Hisada, Emoto, Suzuki, & Okazaki. (2019b, April 17). *Aerobic Exercise Training with Brisk Walking Increases Intestinal Bacteroides in Healthy Elderly Women.* Nutrients, 11(4), 868. https://doi.org/10.3390/nu11040868

News-Medical. (2019, September 25). *Americans still eat too many low-quality carbs and saturated fats, say experts.* News-Medical.net. https://www.news-medical.net/news/20190925/Americans-still-eat-too-many-low-quality-carbs-and-saturated-fats-say-experts.aspx

Paddock, C. (2015, July 13). *Americans "not eating enough fruits and vegetables."* Medicalnewstoday.com; Medical News Today. https://www.medicalnewstoday.com/articles/296677

Quinn, C. (2016, August 12). *A Simple Strategy That'll Make You Drink More Water Every Day.* Thrillist; Thrillist. https://www.thrillist.com/health/nation/hydration-tips-to-drink-more-water-every-day

Shan, Z., Rehm, C. D., Rogers, G., Ruan, M., Wang, D. D., Hu, F. B., Mozaffarian, D., Zhang, F. F., & Bhupathiraju, S. N. (2019, September 24). *Trends in Dietary Carbohydrate, Protein, and Fat Intake and*

Diet Quality Among US Adults, 1999-2016. JAMA, 322(12), 1178. https://doi.org/10.1001/jama.2019.13771

Sondike, S. B., Copperman, N., & Jacobson, M. S. (2003, March). *Effects of a low-carbohydrate diet on weight loss and cardiovascular risk factor in overweight adolescents.* The Journal of Pediatrics, 142(3), 253–258. https://doi.org/10.1067/mpd.2003.4

Stookey, J. D., Constant, F., Popkin, B. M., & Gardner, C. D. (2008, November 16). *Drinking Water Is Associated With Weight Loss in Overweight Dieting Women Independent of Diet and Activity.* Obesity, 16(11), 2481–2488. https://doi.org/10.1038/oby.2008.409

Tantawy, S., Kamel, D., Abdel-Basset, W., & Elgohary, H. (2017a, December 14). *Effects of a proposed physical activity and diet control to manage constipation in middle-aged obese women.* Diabetes, Metabolic Syndrome and Obesity: Targets and Therapy, Volume 10, 513–519. https://doi.org/10.2147/dmso.s140250

Tantawy, S., Kamel, D., Abdel-Basset, W., & Elgohary, H. (2017b, December 14). *Effects of a proposed physical activity and diet control to manage constipation in middle-aged obese women.* Diabetes, Metabolic Syndrome and Obesity: Targets and Therapy, Volume 10, 513–519. https://doi.org/10.2147/dmso.s140250

The technique that will allow us to change the habits we do not like (Charles Duhigg) | Part B' (2022, January 21). Lectures Bureau.

https://www.lecturesbureau.gr/1/the-technique-t
hat-will-allow-us-to-change-the-habits-we-do-not-
like-part-b-2818b/?lang=en

Thornton, S. N. (2016, June 10). *Increased Hydration Can Be Associated with Weight Loss.* Frontiers in Nutrition, 3. https://doi.org/10.3389/fnut.2016.00018

Vij, V. A. (2013, September 7). *Effect of "Water Induced Thermogenesis" on Body Weight, Body Mass Index and Body Composition of Overweight Subjects.* Journal of Clinical and Diagnostic Research. https://doi.org/10.7860/jcdr/2013/5862.3344

Voroshilov, A. P. (2017, May 12). *Modified Qigong breathing exercise for reducing the sense of hunger on an empty stomach* - Alexander P. Voroshilov, Alex A. Volinsky, Zhixin Wang, Elena V. Marchenko, 2017. Journal of Evidence-Based Complementary & Alternative Medicine. https://journals.sagepub.com/doi/10.1177/2156 587217707143#:~:text=The%20Modified%20Qi gong%20Breathing%20Exercise&text=Hold%20 your%20breath%20for%203,Repeat%20this%20e xercise%2010%20times.

Weigle. (2005, July). *A high-protein diet induces sustained reductions in appetite, ad libitum caloric intake, and body weight despite compensatory changes in diurnal plasma leptin and ghrelin concentrations.* The American Journal of Clinical Nutrition, 82(1). https://doi.org/10.1093/ajcn.82.1.41

Wempen, K. (2022, April 29). *Are you getting too much protein?* Mayo Clinic Health System; Mayo Clinic Health System.

https://www.mayoclinichealthsystem.org/hometo
wn-health/speaking-of-health/are-you-getting-too
-much-protein

Yong, M.-S., Lee, Y.-S., & Lee, H.-Y. (2018a, September 30). *Effects of breathing exercises on resting metabolic rate and maximal oxygen uptake.* Journal of Physical Therapy Science, 30(9), 1173–1175. https://doi.org/10.1589/jpts.30.1173

Yong, M.-S., Lee, Y.-S., & Lee, H.-Y. (2018b, September 30). Effects of breathing exercises on resting metabolic rate and maximal oxygen uptake. Journal of Physical Therapy Science, 30(9), 1173–1175. https://doi.org/10.1589/jpts.30.1173

www.ingramcontent.com/pod-product-compliance
Lightning Source LLC
Chambersburg PA
CBHW022058020426
42335CB00012B/746